Dr. Pyke's Natural Way to Complete Stomach Relief

Great Foods and Holistic Methods to Cure Your Upper Digestive Tract Forever

Rob Pyke, M.D., Ph.D.

Prentice Hall Press

Library of Congress Cataloging-in-Publication Data

Pyke, Rob.
  Dr. Pyke's natural way to complete stomach relief : great foods and holistic methods to cure your upper digestive tract forever / Rob Pyke.
     p. cm.
  Includes bibliographical references and index.
  ISBN 0-7352-0298-2 (cloth)
     1. Indigestion—Popular works. 2. Stomach—Diseases—Popular works.
  I. Title: Doctor Pyke's natural way to complete stomach relief. II. Title: Natural way to complete stomach relief. III. Title.

  RC827 .P95 2001
  616.3'32—dc21   2001033231

Acquisitions Editor: *Ed Claflin*
Production Editor: *Tom Curtin*
Interior Design/Page Layout: *Dimitra Coroneos*

© *2001 by* Prentice Hall

Printed in the United States of America

10 9 8 7 6 5 4 3 2 1

ISBN 0-7352-0298-2

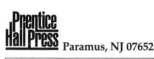 Paramus, NJ 07652

http://www.phdirect.com

Contents

iii

Part 4

MORE ON MEDICINE   *235*

$\mathcal{I}$NTRODUCTION

STOMACH UPSETS: WHAT'S THAT RUMBLING?

Acid stomach distress—dyspepsia—bothers most of us.

A whopping 60 percent of us are prone to a range of four upper gastrointestinal problems. In fact, these four problems are so common that they could be called HUGE (for heartburn, ulcer, gastritis, and esophagitis).

Judging from the ads you see, you might think you can treat any kind of stomach upset with an over-the-counter medication. And most of us swallow the advertising. Only about 10 percent of Americans see a doctor for stomach distress.

Now, maybe you just have an upset stomach, and that's all. But there's a chance that something more serious is causing your gastrointestinal distress. Chronic heartburn produces inflammation of the esophagus (esophagitis). In its most chronic form, it's known as Gastroesophageal Reflux Disease (GERD). This can lead to a highly malignant form of cancer. Erosive gastritis and peptic ulcer often eat deeply enough into the stomach lining to cause fatal bleeding. (Before potent, revolutionary medical treatments became available in the 1970s, the complications of peptic ulcer used to kill 10,000 Americans a year.)

So this book does have a medical section, and in that section, Part 4, I'll describe exactly what these diseases are, how they feel, what causes them, the first line of defense used by doctors. The rest of the book is devoted to things that you can do—that is, a complete nutritional program along with day-to-day lifestyle management advice.

Interestingly enough, the program that heals the stomach will also help prevent another set of chronic diseases: cardiovascular illness. So in the process of healing your stomach, you may also be protecting your heart.

ℚ CLASSIC EXAMPLE OF DYSPEPSIA: ME

I was highly motivated to write this book because I've been a patient myself, and not always a good one.

Most people who know me consider me pretty laid-back—for a doctor. I'm a hard worker, but easy enough to get along with, and I can usually accept change. I say this not to flatter myself, but to point out that I was not an obvious candidate for stress-related illness.

In 1994, I discovered exactly what it's like to experience debilitating stomach trouble. I had just made a move to a different city and had taken on a new job when my health started to go downhill. Six weeks after the move, I developed both stomach and heart trouble. I knew that stress was a factor. But I also observed that my stomach problems got worse when I began taking a new medication prescribed by a cardiologist. I developed a condition known as severe chronic erosive gastritis, which means I was developing hundreds of little holes along my stomach lining.

I also had gastroesophageal reflux disease (GERD) with heartburn and difficulty swallowing. GERD is what you get when the valve between the esophagus and the stomach (called the Lower Esophageal Sphincter, or LES) doesn't keep a tight clamp on the stomach contents. Highly acidic, partially digested food from the stomach backs up through that trapdoor-like valve and lingers in the lower esophagus. The intensely acidic backwash (called reflux) begins to damage the esophageal lining.

The symptoms of GERD were uncomfortable. I had the painful sensation, commonly called heartburn, that results from the "burning" of the reflux gnawing at the esophagus. And I even had trouble swallowing, which means the LES wasn't working right when the food was on its way down. For these problems, an H_2 acid blocker is usually prescribed; in my case, the medication didn't help. Neither did a treatment called dilation of the esophagus, which has been effective for some other patients. Even when I switched cardiac medicines, the result was the same—no relief.

I finally realized that I was limiting my own recovery. I was a passive patient, just "doing what the doctor told me." If I really wanted to get better, I'd have to discover the root problems that were helping to create this stomach discomfort. I decided to take charge of my own lifestyle and diet while continuing to work with the cardiologist and a gastroenterologist.

𝒯AKING CHARGE

Before I did anything else, I thoroughly reviewed the latest findings about nutritional approaches to help the stomach and the heart. The next step, I determined, would be to create stomach-soothing recipes, even if that took trial and error.

Third, I would restart my own program of stress management. Last, I would explore the use of herbal supplements to help wean my stomach from prescription medications.

So here I was, an internist and clinical pharmacologist, looking for a way to get away from prescribed medications in order to heal myself. I realized I was looking for a holistic approach. If a vast array of pharmaceutical medications couldn't heal my stomach, maybe I could succeed in healing it myself, in my own way, with this unique approach that I developed for myself. And if that approach worked for me, perhaps it could work for anyone.

Six months later, my symptoms were gone. I was virtually pain-free. I had truly healed myself, and I was convinced that the holistic approach that worked for me could also work for others.

That is the promise of this book—to help you develop a holistic, self-healing approach to stomach problems. I'd like to help you discover what you can do for yourself and for your own good stomach health, well beyond what your doctor can provide.

I should add that this book is no diatribe against medicine. Far from it. During the six months that I was in recovery, there were many times when I took the prescription drug Prilosec. I would not have wanted to do without it. Nor would I ask you to violate your doctor's orders. What I am asking you to do is to *make yourself a healthy person*.

If that's your goal as well—and I'm sure it seems reasonable enough—then you can't just limp from one dose of medicine to the next, hoping that all these medications will eventually free you from stomach problems. In fact, you may never be able to ignore your stomach again, as you may have done up till now. "Eat like a kid again!" is *not* my rallying cry. Denial won't help you to discover what your stomach has been trying to tell you.

Instead, the approach that you take to heal your stomach may spell out some improvements for your entire lifestyle. As you embrace your newly-felt obligation to yourself, you may eventually become *glad* that you developed a stomach problem because of how much happier you are while practicing healthy ways to live.

ᐂHAT'S IN THIS BOOK FOR YOU?

First, I'll help you figure out whether you have a condition that requires close monitoring and medical treatment. On page 4 you'll find "Who Really Needs to See a Doctor?" Review the self-evaluation to determine if you need more information about medical tests and evaluations. If you do, turn to Part 4, starting on page 235. There, you'll find some practical advice on how to get a proper medical diagnosis, which is necessary before you begin any kind of self-treatment. That way, you can be sure the self-treatment steps that you take are the very best for you.

In Part 1, Lifestyle Changes That Heal Your Stomach, you'll find the basics of lifestyle management and nutritional principles. I'll help you get acquainted with some common dietary offenders, and you'll learn some easy ways to avoid them.

By the time you've finished Part 1, I hope you will be convinced to start eating five small, stomach-healthy meals a day (instead of two or three oversize meals). I'll also guide you toward drinking the right beverages. You'll discover the various forms of exercise, sleeping habits, herbal remedies, and food supplements that can help, and I'll list the top-ten foods and beverages to avoid.

Part 2, Applying Nutritional Principles, lays the groundwork for a healthy, scientific approach to curing your stomach. We now realize that carbohydrate intake is *not* the way to better health, as I'll explain, and why the high glycemic index of all carbohydrates (even the complex ones) produces rebound hunger. But no-fat eating isn't the answer, either—it produces hunger, dissatisfaction, nutrient deficiencies, and even gallstones. Instead, you'll learn about the benefits of the good fats in a low-fat diet, especially the attributes of linoleic and alpha-linolenic acid.

Part 3, Eating Right for a Healthy Stomach, starts with a guide to help you make choices in the supermarket and select the foods to bring home. I'll recommend specific meats, fish, dairy products, oils, nuts, seeds, sauces, vinegars, fruits and vegetables, grains and cereals. And I'll describe snacks that will give your stomach some high-protein comfort.

In the section on beverages, you'll find out which ones may give you stomach pain or gastroesophageal reflux; and I'll recommend various hot and cold beverages for refreshment and enjoyment.

In Part 3 you'll find many recipes from the simple to the exotic for Americanized, fast-cooking, highly nutritious, and digestible meals. You'll even find delicious desserts. (Yes, you can still enjoy cookies, pies, cobblers, crisps, cakes, and frozen and fruity desserts. Each recipe keeps the fat calories below 20%, but none skimps on taste.)

Part 4, More on Medicine, details in plain English how doctors diagnose stomach symptoms, how they treat stomach distress, and what drugs and supplements cause stomach problems or help them.

Finally, Sources and Resources is a compilation of books, articles, and Web sites that I recommend.

ℒIKE TO EAT?

Three principles guided me in developing the recipes found in Part 3. I hope these same principles will inspire you to turn to this section when you're ready to cook up a storm and enjoy some really delicious meals.

1. Cooking for a touchy stomach doesn't mean you must give up flavor. If you've ever been on a "restricted diet," it may have seemed as if the list of foods to avoid included every food you could possibly enjoy. Often, doctors tell us to avoid citrus fruit, citrus juice, cream, margarine, and butter. We're supposed to stay away from tomatoes and tomato products, which eliminates many kinds of foods including pizza, spaghetti, chili, even ketchup. Oh, and peanut butter is out, and you're not supposed to use oils or salad dressings.

So, what's left? Well, many of these lists tell us to exclude cream sauces, fried foods, gravy, fatty meats, peppers of all kinds, and onions. Also proscribed are alcoholic beverages, carbonated beverages, coffee, and cocoa. Last but not least, we're to avoid chocolate, pastries, nuts, spearmint, and peppermint—which means desserts are done for.

Bon appetit—on bread and water!

In my view, such restrictive lists are counterproductive. When there are so many foods we're not supposed to eat, of course we cheat. Then we take pills to counteract our cheating. And still we suffer.

This book shows that it need not be that way. You can enjoy what you eat and still be kind to your stomach! This book presents recipe after recipe of stomach-tested dishes that are tasty rather than boring, and interesting but not excessively exotic.

However, it won't do you any long-term good to eat food that is stomach-healthy and not heart-healthy. That takes us to the second principle:

2. You can cook for stomach health and for heart health, too. There are ways to get what you want and need, without substituting a lot of unfamiliar foods for plain, old-fashioned flavors. I'll give you recipes that meet a double standard, helping your heart while they appeal to your stomach as well.

3. Cooking need not be difficult. To get the "right" diet, you might think that you either have to slave over a stove all day or settle for warmed-up, commercial frozen dishes. But that's not so. It's quite possible for an ordinary person to cook a delicious and healthful meal in a reasonable amount of time. There's no great secret, and you don't have to attend cooking school! Most good, basic meals can be made from scratch in half an hour or less.

You don't need a lot of specialized equipment or ingredients. Every recipe in this book can be prepared with a normal stove, oven, and microwave, and with standard pots and pans.

𝒯HE TEST KITCHEN—ME!

Every recipe in this book was tested on a very tough critic with a very sensitive stomach—me. A recipe is not included in this book unless I liked it and my stomach tolerated it. In the recipes in Part 3, you'll find that I've labeled any ingredients that might create stomach problems, and included suggestions on substitutes for those ingredients.

Feel free to use these recipes as springboards for your imagination. Many people dislike following directions slavishly. The proportions of ingredients always have value as guideposts, but free substitution works as well here as in pro football. The identity of the vegetables, for instance, is easily switched and should depend more on what's in your refrigerator than what's in the original recipe. Ditto for the meats, and remember that you'll do your heart a favor every time you substitute firm tofu or tempeh for meat.

Oh, sure, too many sweet vegetables can make a dish taste weird (see Cooking Chinese), and salty meats like turkey Canadian bacon need to be used sparingly. But remember, there are only two terrible mistakes in cooking: using stale (or spoiled) ingredients and over-cooking.

Five years after my own stomach saga began, I'm not only down to eating three meals a day, I'm also doing vigorous aerobics, I eat an occasional citrus fruit or tomato product, and I can even have a glass of wine once in a while with no distress. So there's hope!

Part 1

LIFESTYLE CHANGES THAT HEAL YOUR STOMACH

Chapter 1

Managing
YOUR
EATING HABITS

If you have any kind of chronic stomach problems, see a doctor. Pain in the upper part of the stomach, or heartburn, could indicate a serious disease—ulcer or gastroestophageal reflux disease. Both of these diseases require a doctor's attention.

When I refer to "chronic," I mean the kind of stomach symptoms that last for an hour, twice a week or more. Also, if you get dyspepsia, or "stomach upset," when you're taking anti-inflammatory drugs, you may have serious stomach problems that call for a doctor's attention.

You also need a doctor if you have symptoms such as weight loss, trouble swallowing, or anemia. Patients older than 45 years with new dyspepsia also need a doctor's workup.

The reason you should see a doctor is that these illnesses might lead to bleeding, perforation, or even cancer. Some of the most serious complications, such as stomach and esophageal cancers, need to be discovered as early as possible. Needless to say, none of us likes to think about such problems. But better to find them earlier rather than later.

Pain that is relieved by eating usually indicates Peptic Ulcer Disease. Again, the doctor can help. Ulcers are better cured with antibiotics than with anything else, but may require a combination of medical treatments. Stress management may also help over the long term.

But stomach pain isn't always caused by ulcer. You may have self-limited symptoms—no disease at all. If you're a smoker, those cigarettes might be to blame. Pain relievers can cause stomach upset, and so can lifestyle habits.

3

Dyspepsia and its associated pain don't always lead to inflammation. Heartburn may simply be heartburn, as long as it does not recur frequently. This is called *functional dyspepsia,* meaning that there is no discernible lesion.

***

WHO REALLY NEEDS TO SEE A DOCTOR?

If you have any kind of chronic stomach problems (dyspepsia), see a doctor. Heartburn or pain in the upper part of the stomach could indicate a serious disease—ulcer or gastroesophageal reflux disease. Both of these diseases require a doctor's attention.

By "chronic," I mean the kind of stomach symptoms that last for an hour, twice a week or more. Also, if you get dyspepsia or "stomach upset" when you're taking anti-inflammatory drugs, you may have serious stomach problems that call for a doctor's attention.

If you're wondering whether you need to see a doctor, the answer is "Definitely" if you have moderate to severe stomach problems. These include the following:

- The problem is frequent: It lasts more than an hour, twice a week.

- It occurs while you are on an anti-inflammatory drug (any pain reliever other than Tylenol).

- It's relieved by eating.

- It comes with an alarm symptom:
  - weight loss,
  - trouble swallowing,
  - anemia,
  - worse pain after eating,
  - belly tenderness, or
  - bleeding.

- It's new or getting worse and you're over 45.

- You are vomiting.

- You have lack of appetite.

For a complete overview of the treatments that doctors offer for various kinds of gastrointestinal (GI) problems, see Part 4, More on Medicine, beginning on page 235.

IMPROPER CONTRACTIONS

Another group of functional (no-disease) symptoms is due to improper contractions of the stomach. This includes vomiting, nausea, flatulence, loss of appetite, and early satiety—feeling full after an abnormally small meal. Bloating, an uncomfortable feeling of fullness, may also suggest no-disease dyspepsia.

On the other hand, you can't always assume that a worse or more frequent kind of discomfort is from the same old mild stomach ailment you have always had. Some ulcers are malignant rather than benign. So are some swallowing difficulties. And many a belly pain comes from an organ other than the stomach. So you need an expert diagnosis first. That way, you can start self-help measures that will help you, rather than hurt you. And you'll find out right away whether you might need surgery or prescription medication, either before or after you make the lifestyle changes and implement the self-help changes that I recommend in my plan.

LIFESTYLE MANAGEMENT

When Americans face self-treatment, their usual approach is to ask what pill or supplement they can take—without changing what they do. Since the dawn of the age of "miracle drugs" with the introduction of cortisone and antibiotics in the 1940s, the culture has encouraged this attitude.

For dyspepsia of all kinds, that attitude can only have limited benefits. Even physicians, formerly the most steadfast adherents to medications and surgery as the cure-alls for diagnosable illnesses, nowadays prescribe such a range of changes in eating, drinking, exercise, and other behavior that they can only be called lifestyle management. Holistic practitioners, of course, see such behavior issues as the *main* focus in treatment of dyspepsia.

Part of lifestyle management is dealing with our self-indulgences, such as smoking, use of alcohol, overstimulation, workaholism, and sedentary, entertainment-filled evenings and weekends.

It's necessary to avoid nicotine and alcohol because they are well proven to cause various kinds of dyspepsia. It's a boon for all kinds of dyspepsia to practice stress management because of the intimate connection between the central nervous system and the gut. We have over a hundred million nerve cells in the gut, a system so organized that it's been called "the second brain."

It's helpful to exercise, no matter what the cause of dyspepsia, to help manage stress, to improve digestive motility, and to optimize body weight.

Of all these lifestyle factors, eating and drinking relate most clearly to our intestinal health. Eating and drinking are also the make-or-break factors in the cure or continuation of dyspepsia.

Here are some basic guidelines to help you manage the lifestyle factors that can make a real difference to your gastrointestinal health.

Identify your dietary offenders and avoid them. The principle is the same, whether your conditions are as mild as simple heartburn or as problematic as peptic ulcer. It's necessary to identify the foods that produce symptoms and avoid them, whether the dyspepsia is related to hyperacidity or not.

To see some of the chief offenders, see the lists on page 29. Remember, these lists suggest only some of the culprits that may be causing trouble. Treat yourself as a special individual. Eat simply at first, until you've identified the chief offenders. Though some foods may be right for other people, that doesn't mean they're right for you. Consulting food lists is no substitute for trial-and-error and personal judgment.

To identify what irritates your own stomach, begin with two or three items per meal. Then gradually add more kinds of food at subsequent meals, until you know what your particular offenders are.

You'll probably know in an hour or two what gives you distress. Be patient with your stomach.

Eat smaller meals. The less food you eat, the less acid it causes and the easier it is to digest. Healing your stomach is worth the self-attention and self-assertion that eating lightly requires, especially in restaurants.

When you eat a smaller meal, the stomach can grind it to a fine pulp and the small intestine can digest it fully. If your stomach has a motility problem—that is, the food moves too slowly as it passes through—eating smaller meals will also help you out. With less of a mechanical job to do, your stomach and small intestine can cope better.

Small meals result in less stomach acid. (Often, the main problem is hyperacidity.) Likewise, the less the meal stimulates the stomach to produce acid, the less acid it will produce after the food has passed through your stomach and entered the small intestine.

That "whoops—too late!" acid flow is called rebound hyperacidity, and it tends to cause dyspepsia about an hour after a meal.

When you eat small meals, you also help to avoid reflux, which is what happens when food and stomach acid "burp up" into the esophagus. Reflux into the esophagus is bad news because it can cause heartburn, inflammation, and even scarring and constriction. In fact, that up-flow, or reflux, is usually not from active muscle contractions (like vomiting) at all. It's backwash, slop-over, just like spilling water when carrying a bucket filled to the brim. Less in the bucket means less slop-over. Less in the stomach means less reflux.

Eating small meals also has other benefits. When you eat a small meal—that is, no larger than 250 calories—you reduce insulin secretion. Insulin is the body chemical that regulates the way your cells use blood sugar for energy. When you have a lot of insulin in your system, you're more likely to have rebound hunger, which can lead to weight gain.

Big meals cause big insulin-gain, leading to greater appetite. In experiments with animals, scientists found that animals that grazed all the time—that is, ate "small meals"—tended to weigh less and live longer than other animals that were restricted to three feedings a day.

Drink less. Pursuing the spillover idea some more, keep in mind that no amount of food restriction will help much if you pour down the fluids with meals. A carried bucket that's half-full of stones doesn't spill easily. But fill it to the brim with water, and soon you'll have a problem with slop-over.

What's more, the larger the liquid volume, the more diluted are the digestive enzymes in it. This slows and limits digestion. Enzymes are catalysts, submicroscopic "grinders" that pursue specific food components and grind them down into simple molecules that the intestine can absorb. If you have a lot of liquids in the mix, the enzymes will be more dilute. The more dilute they are, the fewer the food molecules they can catch and grind.

If you limit your fluid intake during meals, you will also chew your food more thoroughly and eat more slowly, because it takes longer for your salivary glands to moisten the food. This way of eating thus aids your stomach directly.

In general, I advise people to avoid drinking fluids around mealtimes. For half an hour before meals, don't have more than a cup of fluids; and drink as little as possible for an hour or two after the meal. It takes time for your stomach to absorb even plain water.

Modulate your meals. Here are some general guidelines that will help you begin to limit your meals.

At breakfast, have a modest serving each of a high-protein food, a fruit, and a cereal-based side dish. If you're used to eating two or three eggs, have just one, or have half a cup of tofu scramble. Instead of having any eggs at all, eat a breakfast-sized portion of lean meat or fish, accompanied by a slice of toast or half a bagel. Then add a piece of fruit, a small bowl of berries, or a glass of nonacidic fruit juice, and you have a balanced yet small meal.

For lunch, a bowl of soup probably won't be more than 250 calories, as long as it's a non-cream soup. Or have half a sandwich made with lean meat, low-fat cheese, or vegetables. As long as you hold the mayo, butter, and margarine, the half-sandwich is likely to be less than 250 calories.

The size of a dinner at home is easy enough to control. Cook all you please, but limit the portions of everything that you put on your plate. Keep your high-protein dish down to 3 ounces, about the size of a deck of playing cards, whether it's meat, fish, or a bean-based dish. Limit your starch to a couple of ounces dry-weight—the equivalent of a medium potato or one cup of cooked pasta or rice. Limit your vegetable intake to a couple of small dishes, half-cup size. Calories aren't a great concern with vegetables, of course, but you don't need the bulk. If you eat too much, you could be overfilling your stomach.

Whatever you have for dinner, wait an hour or more before you have dessert.

Watch your table time. *How* you eat can be almost as important as *what* you eat. Chew enough so that you don't need to wash your food down. Take 15 to 30 minutes to eat each meal. Pay attention to your food and enjoy it.

The stressful way to eat is to do a second or third activity at the same time you're eating. If you watch TV, read, or even have an intense conversation while you're eating, you're not likely to pay much attention to the way you feel while you're eating. When there's a lot of activity going on, your esophagus and stomach are likely to be pre-stressed before the food and acid arrive in your digestive tract.

Many people with GERD simply don't chew enough. When that happens, bigger pieces of food go to the stomach, prolonging the stomach's task of grinding the food to a liquid. The stomach is slow to empty, holds more gas, and becomes distended.

But there's another side effect of rapid chewing: Less saliva gets mixed with the food. Before the food has been digested, stomach juices start to act on it. That preemptive strike impairs digestion.

In addition, when you chew too little, the pace of your eating obviously speeds up. This, too, is bad for GERD. It tends to make us eat too much, followed rather suddenly by the feeling that we're overly full. There's increased pressure in the stomach, increasing reflux and eventually, when the stomach contents have been acidified, heartburn.

Ordinarily, when you take time to eat slowly, you get a more pleasant feeling of satisfaction from your meal. If you don't allow time, you're already gulping down more food while the signal that says "Enough! You're full!" is still in transit to your brain. So, if you're a fast eater, you essentially overshoot the mark. You end up eating more than is actually required to produce satiety.

So, pay attention to your food. Enjoy it. Put your fork down after a few bites. Pick up your glass and sip a little water. It makes the next bite of food more tasty.

Eating can be tranquil, pleasant, a veritable meditation. Give the food time to help you *feel* full when you *are* full.

STOP THE SPREAD

A fat abdomen impairs stomach function. The only way to counteract this is to lose weight. That requires developing new eating habits, not crash dieting.

Being overweight challenges the valve between the stomach and the intestine (the LES) in several ways. A thick, heavy layer of fat around the outside of the abdomen increases the pressure in the stomach by straining the skin, constricting the amount of volume available to the stomach, and by weighing down on the stomach when you're lying on your back.

But fat doesn't only develop around the outside of the abdomen. It also gets deposited, in similarly large quantities, inside the abdominal cavity, along the intestines. Some men make the mistake of thinking that they can remain overweight but exercise their abdominal muscles enough to harden them. But the hard, external surface of the belly isn't the only part that matters. The internal fat can still contribute to GERD.

I'm sure I don't need to remind anybody that losing weight is a difficult challenge in the culture we live in. One of the best secrets

Watch out when you dine out. If you're dining out, it's usually a lot more difficult to limit the size of your meals. The number-one fear of restaurant owners is that you might leave their establishment feeling cheated—not on price, but because you didn't get enough to eat.

There are two ways to cope with this: 1) the divide-and-conquer approach, and 2) ordering from odd places on the menu.

To divide and conquer, go ahead and order a full, sensible meal. When it's brought to your table, don't dig right in. First, size up your servings. Are these the portions you would take if you were eating at home?

Using your home meals as a rough guide, ruthlessly cut your entire meal into reasonable portions. Take exactly how much you want in is summed up in the simple phrase (which also happens to be the title of a favorite book) *Habits—Not Diets!*

Your eating habits over the long haul will ultimately determine your weight. The best results don't come from any crash diet, diet system, or diet plan. *All* diet plans tend to fail within 6 to 12 months, because the dieter returns to his or her former bad eating habits.

Thinking about habits instead of diets will get you started in the right direction. The vital first step is to keep a diary of everything you eat and drink during the course of a week. With diary in hand, see a dietitian to get one-on-one help. That's especially important if you have any cardiac risk factors. See your doctor *before* you embark on any weight-loss program.

Cardiac risk factors are:

- ❐ You have a history of heart problems.
- ❐ You're male and over forty, or you're female and postmenopausal.
- ❐ You have high blood pressure, diabetes, or high cholesterol;
- ❐ Other people in your family have had cardiac problems before they reached the age of 60;
- ❐ You smoke.

each dish, then shove anything that's left over to the far side of the plate or bowl.

Would that embarrass you? You're not an oddball if you simply don't need the "leftovers." You're someone who is health-oriented and takes charge of your own life.

The other way to deal with those waiters trying to ply you with calories at the restaurant is to skip the "dinners" and "entrees" sections of the menu entirely. Order instead from the lists of appetizers, salads, soups, and side dishes. Ask about half portions, or find out whether you can have the child-size portion. Don't worry; nowadays, all restaurants are accustomed to discriminating diners who do this.

For frequent feedings, bring food with you. Who has time to make five or six meals a day? Obviously, that would mean a lot of time in the kitchen. Most of us can't even get away from chores or the desk for a mid-morning snack or mid-afternoon break.

But there are ways to make your in-between meals a lot easier. With the half-bagel left from your morning breakfast, you have the makings of a perfect mid-morning snack. Slather it with a high-protein or fruity spread (you'll find a recipe on page 128), wrap it, and bring it to work with you. That will be your second small feeding of the day. Alternatively, be a stress-fighter who combines time-management with time-outs: Go to the kitchen or the cafeteria and get a similar snack in mid-morning.

In the mid-afternoon, have a piece of fruit along with the half of the sandwich you saved from lunch. Take time between phone calls and chores, or when someone else is talking at a meeting, to refresh yourself.

In the evening, have your small dinner early, at least four hours before bedtime. Two hours later, you will have the appetite for a snack—and that's still another two hours before you go to bed.

Enjoy your low-fat meals, along with other foods. In Part 2, Applying Nutritional Principles, you'll find plenty of information about the many benefits of low-fat eating. Just so you know, I'm not going to advocate draconian measures that only allow 10 percent fat in your diet. Such diets do exist, precluding the consumption of nearly all meat, cheese, eggs, oils, and nuts. But those extreme levels of restriction are neither necessary nor optimal for a healthy stomach. They can even cause new health problems.

Instead, the goal of this program is to limit your intake of dietary fat to a moderate 20 percent of your daily calories. This is much less than the 30 to 40 percent fat diet that most Americans eat, but it's not so drastic that it deprives your body of the fat it needs.

At this level of fat restriction, your hormonal system can still function normally, and that's essential, since your hormonal system is integrally connected to digestion. By following the fat guidelines described here, you'll be adapting a diet that has highly beneficial effects. It slows gastric emptying, reduces reflux esophagitis, and helps prevent heartburn.

Opt for low-acid meals. If you eat a lot of sour foods or drink quantities of coffee, you raise the total acidity in your body. That worsens dyspepsia. So if you're prone to acid stomach, sour food and coffee are two things you need to avoid.

What is a low-acid meal? Maybe we should start with some definitions. Chemists measure acidity in terms of the solutions of acid in water. Their measuring stick is called *pH* (just say "pee-aitch.") It's a mathematical term, not an abbreviation.

If a substance has a pH of 0, it's about as acidic as anything can get. (Technically, it's possible to get down to a minus one, but that's acid so concentrated that it burns the skin in seconds.) As the numbers climb up the pH scale, the balance between acid and its opposite, alkaline, comes closer and closer to reaching exact equivalency. When the pH is 7, the substance is perfectly neutral. That is, acidity and alkalinity are balanced out.

Coming down from the neutral pH of 7, every decrease of one point means ten times as much free acidity per unit of volume. Straight vinegar (5% acetic acid, a weak acid) has a pH around 4, so it's a thousand times more acid than pure, neutral water. The sourness of vinegar is really the taste of acid, but it's not so acidic that it hurts the tongue.

The stomach makes so much strong acid that it keeps the pH around 2 when it's empty. That's about a hundred times more acid than vinegar! This is the lowest pH anywhere in the body, and it's very irritating.

Your stomach puts up with this degree of acidity in two ways. One is by secreting a thick, adherent layer of mucus that protects it. The other way, the more enjoyable way, is by becoming more alkaline as you eat your small, frequent meals during the day. As soon as you put a meal of neutral foods in your stomach, the pH rises to around 4.

The more acid that goes in with food, the lower it drives the pH down—the stronger the acid, that is. Of course, a little acidity doesn't make much difference. If you squeeze some lemon juice on your fish, that small amount of acid won't matter. But if you decide to have a whole tomato, orange, or grapefruit—all very acidic foods—you're taking on an acid load that will make a difference to your stomach.

The effects are even worse if you take in a large volume of an acidic beverage, as happens when you drink a large cup of coffee (whether it's regular or decaf). Worst of all is a large amount of acid that has been concentrated down, as in tomato sauce.

Later, I'll give you some specific guidelines on low-acid eating, and also some advice on low-acid beverages.

SOME ACID COMMENTS

Any chemist who's reading this will be dissing me by now. I've blurred *active* acidity with *total* acidity. I'd better stop pussyfooting around, because this is important stuff to dyspeptics, not just to chemists.

Stomach acid, hydrochloric acid, is a strong acid. Essentially all of its acidity is free. That's good, because hydrochloric acid needs to be ready to kill any bacteria that reach your stomach.

Hydrochloric acid holds nothing back. That is, there's nothing bound up in its molecular backpack to prevent it from going to work, in full force, in bacteria destruction. Its active acidity is equal to its total acidity.

Vinegar and all the acids found in foods don't work like hydrochloric acid. They're known as weak acids. Just a tiny fraction of their total acid is released if a weak acid is placed in a solution whose pH is between 0 and 4.

Since their total acidity is much greater than their active acidity, they don't taste irritatingly sour, even when concentrated. In fact, you could put pure crystals of citric, tartaric, or ascorbic acid right on your tongue without injury. Even though they're highly acidic, they're the weak acids that don't immediately release all the acid that they hold. Just like tomato sauce, these food acids can release a lot of acid in your body, even though you don't immediately taste the acid on your tongue.

Acetic acid is the strongest of all the acids we eat or drink. Citric and tartaric and the others are all a lot weaker. So when we enjoy a tart grapefruit (pH 5) or other tangy food, we are taking in a huge load of acid. Your intestine is prepared to neutralize the acid that's produced by the stomach; but the acid that comes from grapefruit and other tart foods is far more acidic than the intestine expects.

No bedtime snacking! When you have a snack just before you lie down, you're inviting reflux. If you're too hungry to sleep, have just a small snack and cover it with antacids.

Bedtime snacking is bad for the stomach and the esophagus in two big ways. First, lying down is an invitation to reflux. The LES—that valve at the base of the esophagus that keeps food down in the stomach—can all too easily fail, and it does so regularly if you have heartburn or esophageal reflux disease.

If your stomach is empty, the pH creeps down toward 2, even at night. That's okay if your stomach is nearly empty. If you just have a few tablespoons or less in your stomach, the contents are almost lost in the big stomach bag (which doesn't shrink). But when you have a meal-size load of contents in the stomach, reflux is likely.

Of course, the pH in the stomach is raised by the meal, but that doesn't really help. The stomach contents are irritating when they get outside the stomach, and that's exactly what happens when those contents creep past the LES at the top of your stomach and get into your esophagus. There's immediate irritation, caused by the acid stomach contents coming in contact with other tissue. So don't kid yourself that a bedtime snack (or a middle-of the-night refrigerator raid) is going to help you by buffering your insides.

Suppose it's the middle of the night and you're too hungry to sleep. What should you do?

The way to take care of your stomach and esophagus while you relieve the stomach's annoying contractions (hunger pains) is to have a snack. But I advise you to minimize and cover it.

First of all, minimize the amount of food, and minimize how much you drink. In fact, if you drink anything, make sure it's only a few small sips of fluid.

By "cover," I mean buffering that small amount of food with the only thing that instantly raises the pH out of the irritating range—antacids. It may take a lot of antacids. In fact, you'll need to take four to six of the usual over-the-counter tablets or a full ounce of an antacid liquid to "cover" your snack for even two hours.

If offender foods are unavoidable, minimize your exposure. What if you have dyspepsia and your only options are to go hungry for a long, uncomfortable period of time or to eat something that is probably going to kick up your pain?

You had better act carefully so you don't suffer later. First, make a preemptive strike. Take a dose of antacids or, if you are not taking prescription medication for your stomach already, take an acid-blocker. Then, minimize your exposure.

This is not rocket science, but here are a few ideas to help you avoid acidic condiments:

➡ Scrape as much of the barbecue sauce off the chicken as you can.

➡ Ditto the condiments on the burger.

➡ Skip the cocktail sauce for the shrimp, and substitute a lick of lemon juice.

➡ Dilute the Hunan beef or other spicy main dish in your stomach with potatoes, rice, or other bland starch.

I also recommend that you experiment to find what dietary supplements and herbal preparations can help in these circumstances. Later in the book I'll recommend some specific herbs that are benign to the body and pleasant to take.

Look for foods that will benefit your stomach. Many foods are neutral to the treatment of dyspepsia. They form the bulk of what is recommended in the recipes in Part 3, Eating Right for a Healthy Stomach. A good example is rice. It is very easily digested, so it contributes nothing to gas and cramps and minimizes stomach discomfort.

Another, more complex example is nonfat milk. It buffers stomach acid, providing immediate relief. But even though it helps a lot of people, it might not be right for you. In some people, the stomach responds to the presence of milk (even skim or nonfat milk) by producing more stomach acid than usual. So it may be a mistake to have milk without providing buffering or an antacid within the next hour.

ℒOOSEN YOUR BELT

Any measure that relieves the pressure on the stomach from clothing can help relieve GERD. Stop trying to fit into those too-small pants. Have them let out or wear others that fit loosely around the waist.

If your belt is too tight, simply get a larger belt and let it all the way out. Better yet, wear suspenders instead.

$\mathcal{D}$ON'T STRAIN

Bending forward and straining both cause reflux, so watch the way you exercise. If you perform abdominal exercises, it's a habit to train yourself out of. Such maneuvers squeeze the stomach and defeat the LES. If you do perform abdominal exercises, wait at least three hours after eating before you work out. Even if you've only had some water to drink, you should wait two hours before you do any abdominal exercises.

If you have to lean forward and strain because you're constipated, take some measures to relieve constipation. Start walking half an hour a day, increase your fiber intake, and drink at least two quarts of water a day. These are the best routine ways to become regular and have reasonably soft stools.

If that's not enough, get a laxative. Try taking Metamucil® or another good source of fiber every day. An all-fiber laxative softens stool without cramping the bowel.

The next resort for regular use should be a pharmaceutical stool softener such as Colace® or Dialose®. Or, as needed, you can take a laxative such as milk of magnesia. But avoid laxatives that are spasm-inducing, and ones that contain senna, cascara, or phenolphthalein. Since they are habit-forming, they are the last resort, and should be used only occasionally.

Learn how to belch. People who get that bloated, gassy feeling in the stomach but don't have other options available to unbind their stomachs, or don't have heartburn or GERD, might profit from learning how to belch. This is risky for people with heartburn, because belching opens the LES, allowing reflux. So it's not for everybody. But if it's bloating alone that you need to relieve, belching can help.

Women may say, "Yes, that's easy for you to say—you're a guy! It's socially permissible for you to gross people out."

In defense of my belching advocacy, I can only state that I'm not asking anyone to belch loudly in formal situations. I'm saying that if you learn how to rid yourself of gas without medications or herbals, you are providing yourself with one more tool—one that's free and always accessible—to deal with stomach distress.

When learning to belch, all you need to do is learn to half-swallow a small mouthful of air. That pushes the epiglottis and the lower esophageal sphincter (LES) open, so there's a free passage from the stomach to the mouth. Stop breathing for a couple of seconds, then open your mouth after you make the half-swallow. That lets the gas out.

You don't have to be super-efficient and make one huge belch to relieve the gas. It may take a couple of dozen small belches. You may have to help the effort with a walk, or bounce slightly on your feet, or rhythmically give yourself a little Heimlich maneuver, pushing on the stomach after you open your mouth. Any benign maneuver that puts modest extra pressure on the stomach may help expel the gas. That's all you need to do. But do it standing upright, not sitting or lying down, so you don't push liquid stomach contents into your esophagus.

Walk to soothe your stomach. Moderate exercise, especially walking, aids gastrointestinal motility. But that is only the start of the benefits walking conveys. It also lifts the mood and relieves stress.

Psychiatrists recommend exercise for anxious and depressed patients. One biological psychiatrist who studies the effects of antidepressants estimated that exercise alone conveys about 25 percent of the relief needed to help restore feelings of normalcy in someone who is depressed.

Any kind of repetitive movement, even something as simple as chewing gum, affects the way the chemical serotonin acts within the brain. Elevated serotonin levels contribute to a sense of well-being and relaxation.

Aerobic exercise has an effect on the hormone adrenaline, too. Progressively, over time, exercise raises the adrenaline levels, and this raises one's mood.

I'm not a fan of running, however. Running can *cause* heartburn, even in GERD patients who have not eaten for awhile. Recent research has proven the link. Among the athletes tested were runners, weight lifters, and cyclists. Each waited one hour after eating a small meal, then worked out for an hour. Studies showed that running caused the most acid reflux; weight lifting caused less; and bicycling caused the least. Apparently it's the jostling motion that does it.

Of course, there's another reason not to run (at least in my view), and that's the frequency of injury in runners. Running can strain the heels, ankles, knee joints, and hips. All these joints get jolted and worn with hundreds of pounds of extra pressure each time a runner's foot lands.

Stay upright after eating. All of the instructions for relieving dyspepsia and GERD recommend staying upright for at least two hours after eating. The trouble is, eating can make people feel sleepy. So it is doubly important not to eat large meals: to help an ailing stomach cope with the load, and to help you keep awake until the stomach contents have gone to the intestine. This takes an hour or less after a small snack and about two hours after an ordinary-size meal, but up to five hours after a big feast.

TILT THE BED

By raising the head of your bed a few inches, you can help relieve reflux.

Even if you wait two hours after eating to go to bed, an impaired LES may still spill acidic stomach contents into the esophagus if you sleep on a flat bed. Tilting the head of the bed up helps prevent this. There are various ways to do it.

One way is to cut two short, equal lengths of pipe. Put them under the legs at the head of the bed. If the bed has casters, the casters should fit snugly inside the pieces of pipe so the bed won't wobble around.

As for how high your bed should be, check with your doctor. You'll want to keep the height minimized, because the higher you go, the more you slide toward the foot of the bed and cramp your toes overnight. Your doctor may recommend 4, 6, or even 8 inches.

There's another way to raise the head of your bed. Get a long, tapered wedge of foam plastic at a medical appliance store and put it under your mattress cover. The wedge should be 4 to 8 inches thick at the head end, tapering to zero at the base of the V. Place the wedge so the bottom of the V is at or below your hips. The wedge need be no wider than the space you sleep on, so you can have the wedge under your side of the bed without interfering with the other side. (This is an advantage of the wedge: If your spouse wants a horizontal bed and you need it raised, this arrangement can accommodate both.)

Some people recommend using big wood blocks under the casters at the head of the bed. The drawback to this method is that, if you are restless in bed, the bed could fall off the blocks, giving you a nasty jolt. If the blocks are big enough, this method could work, but using the sections of pipe or the foam wedge is far preferable, in my view.

As for what *not* to do, don't elevate your head only, or your head and chest, with pillows. That squeezes the stomach, worsening the problem instead of relieving it.

TOP FOODS TO HELP PREVENT DYSPEPSIA

Some foods have properties that make them especially beneficial for anyone who has dyspepsia. When you're testing these foods, be cautious at first. Some of them must be used carefully or they can worsen your symptoms. If you have an adverse reaction, just reduce the amount you eat.

FOOD OR BEVERAGE	PROPERTIES THAT HEAL OR PROTECT	DOSING INFORMATION
Yogurt	Probiotic bacteria help:	Cup
Sauerkraut	❑ digest lactose (in all dairy products) thus reducing the gas and bloating;	Individualize; too much can create gas instead of dispelling it.
Miso	❑ digest protein and fat; ❑ speed transit of food; and ❑ reduce the amount of gas produced in the bowel.	
Low-fat soy milk	Buffers stomach acid; slowly digested so protection lasts.	Cup
Artichoke	Higher in fructooligosaccharides among common foods benign to the stomach; nourishes probiotic bacteria.	One
Green juices: barley, alfalfa, wheat	Promote healing directly.	½ cup or less
Papaya	Contain digestive enzymes.	¼ to ½ cup
Pineapple		
Ginger	Stops spasms and cramps.	Individualize; excess worsens symptoms.
Fennel	Relieves pain, dispels gas, relieves overacidity.	

Other worthwhile foods to try for relief of stomach distress include okra and squash. **Okra** is a demulcent food, easing ulcer or gastritis pain because of all the mucinous material inside the green covering. It is reputedly good for many intestinal disorders, also.

Squash can help soothe the stomach. A diet high in squash may also help lower the risk of cancer. The deep orange winter squash, such as butternut and hubbard, are loaded with cancer-fighting carotenoids such as beta-carotene.

Chapter 2

Supplements and Herbs to Help Digestion

While there are no magic pills that can instantly heal your stomach or prevent dyspepsia, a number of supplements and herbs can be helpful. Just be sure, when you're taking them, that you also continue to take the other measures for lifestyle management.

Among the food supplements that can be very effective is **L-glutamine**. This is the beneficial component of cabbage juice, but it comes in supplement form. If you take the pure supplement, have a dose of 500 milligrams of L-glutamine daily, either before meals or several hours after eating.

Pectin has been reported in a controlled study to be an effective supplementation for people who have duodenal ulcers. Pectin comes from apples, especially their skins, and it's a demulcent, which means that it soothes irritation.

I also recommend **Vitamin E**. If you take 400 to 800 IU daily (the IU stands for International Units, a standard measure), you'll reduce stomach acid and alleviate some of the pain it causes. A number of studies suggest that vitamin E has a protective effect, helping to prevent the formation of ulcers in humans and animals. At dosages of 400 to 800 IU daily, vitamin E is nontoxic, and you can take it for years.

Vitamin A at 50,000 IU three times a day for four weeks was shown in two controlled clinical trials to help heal stomach ulcers. One trial was in stress-induced gastric ulcers; the other was in chronic gastric ulcers. No side effects or toxicity appeared in the patients in these two trials. However, excessive Vitamin A intake produces skin discoloration and other major toxicity problems, so this regimen should not be prolonged or followed without professional advice.

Vitamin C deficiency has long been known to cause scurvy, which is characterized by non-healing ulcers of the mucous membranes. In a French study, intravenous supplementation of Vitamin C promoted healing of gastric and duodenal ulcers as quickly as routine medical treatments did.

In case of actual or suspected peptic ulcer, supplementation with Vitamin C would seem prudent. However, plain unbuffered Vitamin C is ascorbic *acid*, a reasonably strong organic acid. It can contribute to stomach irritation when taken in quantities over 250 milligrams a day. So, for safety's sake, take a buffered or ester form of Vitamin C.

Zinc at 50 to 80 milligrams daily promotes quicker healing in general. This dosage cannot be taken for months on end because of likely toxicity, but it's safe to take for a couple of weeks. If you do supplement with zinc, however, be sure to take it with meals, since zinc can cause nausea if you take it on an empty stomach.

Bloating is sometimes a result of replacement of digestion-aiding bacteria in the gut by unfriendly or even toxic bacteria. This is called dysbiosis. You can help prevent it with supplements called **probiotic bacteria** mixes.

Probiotic mixes help recolonize the intestine with lactobacillus acidophilus, bifidobacterium bifidum, and bifidobacterium longum. (On the labels, these names are sometimes listed simply as "lactobacillus and bifidus species.") The helpful bugs suppress disease-promoting bacteria and provide half a dozen other benefits: They promote production of enzymes that help digest protein and fat. They increase passage of food through the gut, relieving constipation. They reduce gas production. They help digest lactose. They make B vitamins. And they suppress the growth of yeast (*Candida albicans*).

The usual dosage is one or two capsules a day. Probiotic bacteria have almost no side effects. In order to be effective, however, the mixture must be stored in a refrigerator or freezer. The good bacteria are fragile.

Fructooligosaccharides (say FRUIK-toe-OL-igo-SAK-a-rides) or **FOS** are natural sugars that pass through the stomach intact. These commercial sweeteners are good for you. They feed and thus stimulate growth of gut-friendly bacteria, working in concert with lactobacillus and bifidus species. They are also avid moisteners, absorbing water. In

FOS capsules, the sugars are often mixed in with lactobacillus and bifidus species. Take one or two a day.

Reading labels for bacterial content is a bit unnerving. It's anybody's guess which species are most beneficial and how many of the three billion or so bacteria that you get in each capsule are actually needed. In fact, you can't even be sure how many of these bacteria survive storage long enough to get into your stomach. So your own experience is the real test.

Try a capsule or two with breakfast every day for a week or two and see how you feel. Gas should diminish or disappear entirely, and stool passage and odor should be more pleasant. If not, start taking a capsule or two with dinner also.

ℋERBAL STOMACH HEALERS

The following suggestions on herbs to relieve dyspepsia are given in collaboration with Barry Sherr, Nutritionist-Clinical Herbalist A.H.G., a prominent herbalist who owns Chamomile Natural Foods in Danbury, CT.

Herbs that heal wounds and ulcers (and guard against bacterial infection) are called vulneraries, and many have been used for centuries—even millennia—for that purpose.

Aloe vera and DGL, a purified form of licorice, are tops among the herbs that can help heal your stomach. Chamomile, ginger, and catnip are other good soothers for stomach aches.

Drinkable **aloe** is available as juices or gels. Irish moss is added as a thickening agent in gels. Gels coat mucous membranes more thickly and last longer. Use aloe as a carrier for all the herbs mentioned in this chapter. Overdoing aloe will soften the stool and have a laxative effect (not unwelcomed events for most Americans). As aloe acts also as a uterine stimulant, it must not be used during pregnancy.

Licorice is probably the strongest herb that's recommended by herbalists for treating stomach upsets or even peptic ulcer. In fact, plain, unprocessed licorice root is *too* strong. If you take it in large quantities, pure licorice has strong hormonal effects. It can make the kidneys retain salt and water while wasting potassium from the body. This weakens all muscles including the heart, causing high blood pressure, congestive heart failure, and even cardiac arrest.

The main culprit among the components of licorice is glycyrrhetinic acid. Removal of this component is called deglycerrhizinating.

Deglycerrhizinated licorice, abbreviated **DGL**, can be found at many health food stores. (One preparation is called CAVED-S.) In controlled studies, this herb has been found as effective as H_2-blockers for healing gastric and duodenal ulcers. It may also protect against aspirin-induced gastric erosions.

At a cellular level, DGL works by regenerating the mucus-secreting cells that form glands along the stomach lining. The stomach's output of mucin increases, providing protection against acid. Usually one or two capsules, taken three times a day, will provide some relief.

NOTE: As licorice has hormonal effects, it must not be used during pregnancy.

Comfrey (*Symphytum officinale*) is a marvelous healer of gastric mucosa. It's important to use tinctures that are labeled "P.A. Free" as the P.A., a Pyrazaline Alkaloid, is a liver irritant. Teas or capsules are not usually P.A. Free and shouldn't be used. The P.A. Free Comfrey tincture promotes granulation, or the closing of a wound by increasing growth of the tissue surrounding it.

Two other foods, **cabbage** and **garlic**, have been used to help heal ulcers. Garnet Cheney, at Stanford Medical School, discovered that cabbage juice could help heal stomach ulcers. He isolated from the juice a substance he calls Vitamin U, which is now sold under the trade names Coboagin-U, Epadyn-U, Vitas-U, and Ardesyl.

Plain **cabbage juice** has more components than the isolated chemicals found in cabbage, and a number of scientists recommend it. Leonard Mervyn, Ph.D., fellow of the Royal Society of Chemistry, discovered the role of coenzyme Q10 in humans. A biochemist and author of a series of health guides including *Stomach Ulcers: Safe Alternatives without Drugs*, Mervyn speculates in his book on natural treatments and diet for peptic ulcers that the high concentrations of Vitamin C and the amino acid glutamine in the juice may also be important components contributing to ulcer healing.

The acidity of cabbage juice, however, may limit the amount that you can tolerate. If you wish to try it, start small, with just an ounce, then slowly increase the dose until you're taking a whole liter over a day, which is slightly more than 4 cups. Of course, if you get more pain rather than less, back off.

Garlic is recommended by Dr. Mervyn as an intestinal antiseptic that may also help eradicate *H. Pylori,* the bacteria that cause gastric ulcers. It may work through its component called allicin, an antiseptic. Because of its peculiar stomach irritant properties, garlic should be tried in its mildest form (roasted) and in small quantities. After you find out how well you tolerate it, you can try the raw clove, allicin-rich garlic extract pills, or full medicinal doses of either. The irritating effects of garlic can be mediated by aloe gel, as mentioned before.

Several herbs contain mucinous substances, even the glue called Mucilage, that soothe where they are applied. Such herbs for oral use are called demulcents. All demulcents need be taken with a full glass of water, so that the dry mucilage and other components are well hydrated and can form a natural, soothing gel in the stomach.

One demulcent is **marshmallow root** (althea or althaea). You can take 2 to 5 grams of dried root three times a day, or 1 teaspoonful of the powdered root infused in a cup of hot water.

Another recommended demulcent is **slippery elm bark (ulmus)**. Place 1 to 2 teaspoonfuls of dried herb in a cup of water, heat the water (to make an infusion), then drink it slowly.

Several fresh herbs are also recommended for stomach problems. **Basil** may prevent stomach ulcers. The recommended dose is 1 teaspoon of crushed leaves steeped for 10 minutes in boiling water. If the sweetness bothers you, add a twist of lemon.

Rosemary may also ease stomach upsets. At least 1 teaspoon of the short, thick needles must be steeped 15 minutes to extract the active principle. (One authority recommends 2 teaspoonfuls.) Alvita offers tea bags of the herb. If you find the taste unpleasant, you can make a mixed infusion by adding other herbs such as chamomile or spearmint for sweetness, or roasted chicory for bitterness.

Chicory works solo, too. The root and leaves contain bitter substances that stimulate the appetite and help ease stomach upsets. The recommended dose is 1 teaspoonful steeped in a cup of hot water for 5 minutes. Use it fresh or dried, but not roasted. (The active compounds are decomposed in the roasting process.)

Peter Rabbit, perhaps the first character in literature who ate and ran—and suffered the stomach consequences—was lucky. The mother of this antihero did the right thing when she gave her naughty bunny a cup of **chamomile tea** after his stressful day at Mr. Magregor's garden. Chamomile soothes the stomach and stops its painful contractions.

The usual dosage (for humans, not rabbits) is 1 or 2 tea bags' worth, steeped for at least 5 minutes in 6 to 8 ounces of hot water straight from a boiling teakettle. Chamomile is also available in capsules that contain the dried flower. Take one or two capsules with a cup of water.

(I prefer the chamomile tea to the dried flower. When the capsules of dry flowers pop open in your stomach, they may add to your nausea for a brief time, starting a couple of minutes after they are swallowed.)

A sufficient amount of chamomile to soothe your stomach may make you drowsy. That's fine, of course, if you're at home and about to fall asleep anyway, but not so fine if you have to get in the car and drive. In that case, try one capsule of chamomile and one capsule of catnip. **Catnip** is a stomach soother on its own, and the combination of both catnip and chamomile seems to work better than either one of them taken alone.

Bayberry, goldenseal root, myrrh, parsley, and **sage** all have some qualities as mucous membrane tonics and stomach-relievers. Bayberry and goldenseal both contain berberine, a genuine antibiotic. If you take 25 to 50 milligrams of berberine, three times a day for two weeks, you can suppress or even eliminate *Candida, H. Pylori*, or more virulent parasites like *Giardia*. But if you're trying to get enough berberine by consuming goldenseal or bayberry, check the berberine content of the herb; it can vary widely.

Anise seeds can stimulate digestion and relieve nausea and flatulence. The recommended dose is 1 teaspoon of the powdered seed made into a tea with a cup of hot water. The volatile oil smells and tastes wonderful, and that oil is actually the active principle. Anisette and other liqueurs containing peppermint were originally produced to help digestion, but that's no reason to favor those liqueurs: The alcohol in them holds no benefit at all.

A WORD OF HERBAL CAUTION

CAUTION: If you are taking medications, consult with your doctor before trying these herbs. Pectin can interfere with tetracycline antibiotics (Achromycin, Sumycin) and with lovastatin (Mevacor). Ginger, Vitamin E, and garlic can interfere with anticoagulants (blood thinners). Ginger and licorice can interfere with medicines for high blood pressure. Aloe and ginger can interfere with some cardiac medicines including antiarrhythmics and digitalis-type drugs; aloe can interfere with diuretics, too. Licorice can interfere with aspirin, NSAIDs, corticosteroids, and other hormone therapy. Finally, garlic, ginger, licorice, and chromium can interfere with antidiabetic drugs.

Chapter 3

$\mathcal{A}$VOID THE STOMACH OFFENDERS

$\mathcal{A}$s I emphasized in Chapter 1, it's important to find out what foods are causing you the most problems. Obviously, people react in unique ways to different foods. The foods in this chapter are the ones that seem to be the most common offenders for people who have intestinal and stomach problems. Some of the worst are the foods you're most likely to eat if you stop for fast food or dine at an unfamiliar restaurant.

Chocolate and fat are both common offenders, but there are many others.

Onion is highly acid and generates more acid when exposed to water. Hamburgers are high on the list because of their high fat content; because beef fat (tallow) is so saturated that it is especially hard to digest; and because they are usually consumed with other offenders such as mayonnaise, pickles, onions, ketchup, and mustard.

Butter, margarine, premium ice cream, and nuts are on the list because they are high-fat foods that weaken the LES. Buffalo wings combine hot pepper with high fat for a one-two punch.

Concentrated tomato products are there because they have concentrated acid. All hot peppers—black, red (cayenne), chilies, Jalapeno, and all the related little vegetable firecrackers—are also offenders, irritating the esophagus and stomach.

FOODS TO AVOID

Want a quick list of foods to re-move from your menu? Here are the top ten.

1. Peppermint
2. Chocolate
3. Onions
4. Hamburgers
5. Butter & margarine
6. Tomato paste or sauce
7. Hot peppers
8. Premium ice cream
9. Nuts
10. Buffalo wings

BEVERAGES TO AVOID

What are the beverages that are most likely to cause dys-pepsia? Here's the top-ten list.

1. Wine
2. Beer
3. Coffee
4. Chocolate
5. Colas
6. Grapefruit juice
7. Orange juice
8. Tomato juice
9. Tea
10. Cocoa

NOTE: It's not the caffeine in coffee and tea that's entirely to blame for kicking up GERD or ulcers. Caffeine does weaken the LES, but the rest of the brew does more harm.

Although I advise people to avoid both coffee and tea, you may be somewhat comforted to learn that tea affects fewer people than coffee does. Many people wonder, however, whether it makes sense to neu-tralize the effects of coffee or tea by adding whole or skim milk. Whole milk causes a much higher incidence of heartburn than skim milk, so I don't recommend it. But adding a jigger of skim milk to tea (or coffee) is less irritating.

30

UPSETS ON THE WAY

Apart from the beverages that are likely to bring on dyspepsia, there are a number that directly cause reflux (which creates heartburn). These include carbonated beverages, citrus juices, and some other kinds of juices. This list shows which fluids can give you heartburn.

FLUID	% REPORTING HEARTBURN
Water	20
Citrus	68–73
Tomato	70
Pineapple	62
Apple, Cranberry, Grape	39–46
Colas, regular	55–57
Colas, diet	49–51
Root beer, lemon-lime sodas	35–38
Beer, red & white wine	60–67
Coffee	79
Tea	57
Whole milk	38
Low-fat milk	28
Skim milk	22

Incidentally, the figure for water isn't just a placebo response. All beverages make the stomach respond with a certain amount of acid production, so even water can provoke real heartburn.

A word about drinking alcohol when you have GERD: Don't. I think anyone with gastrointestinal reflux should simply avoid all alcoholic drinks. Wine and beer are problematic on their own, but on top of the consequences of ingesting alcohol, these beverages are often consumed with a heavy meal in the evening, which increases the chances of reflux.

$\mathcal{D}$ON'T BE TAKEN IN BY TAKE-OUT

When you're on the go and your only alternative is take-out food, you can still help your stomach by making some smart choices about what you eat.

One recent survey found that most of us stop at a fast-food restaurant at least once a week, and nearly a third of us have breakfast "on the go" almost every morning. Since fast food is usually very high in fat, this survey amounts to a national fire alarm for GERD and ulcers.

Is it possible to eat well on the go? Well, maybe. Try these recommendations for good-tasting treats that will help rather than hurt your stomach.

BREAKFAST CAREFULLY

Avoid fast-food places that have only high-fat breakfast dishes such as donuts, greasy sandwiches, and hash browns. You're better off at a bagel place, a deli, or a coffee shop. Dunkin' Donuts has good bagels. Health-food delis and gourmet delis are even better bets. Order a combination of food and drink that will give you protein to buffer your stomach and feed your head; complex carbohydrates to give you energy without rebound hunger; and vitamins and minerals.

Here are some bases, toppings, and juices that I recommend:

BASE	TOPPINGS	JUICES
Whole Wheat or Rye Bagel	Nonfat or low-fat cream cheese*	Grape
Whole Wheat & Raisin English Muffin	Sprinkle olive oil plus low-fat mozzarella, cheddar, or Swiss cheese	Pear
Whole Wheat Pita	Peanut butter*	Peach
Toast—whole wheat, rye, or oatmeal	*To sweeten, add Polaner or Sorrel Ridge all-fruit spread	Apple—last choice because it's virtually all (natural) sugar water

For your hot drink, don't order coffee or decaf. Brew herb tea for yourself: Bring your own tea bags and order hot water. Don't add cream or the coffee whitener. (That whitener is titanium dioxide.)

If you're a newcomer to herb teas, here are some samples that you might want to try:

BITTER	SWEET	TART
Good Earth Green tea blend decaffeinated	Stash Licorice Spice Herbal Tea	Celestial Seasonings Country Peach Passion, Red Zinger, or Lemon Zinger
Caffeine-Free Tea, Good Seasonings Herb Tea	Celestial Seasonings Emperor's Choice	
The Republic of Tea Desert Sage Tea or Tea of Inquiry	The Republic of Tea Moroccan Mint	Alvita Rose Hips or Rosemary (herbal) tea
	Celestial Seasonings Sleepy Time (Probably just at night; it really *does* make you sleepy).	Lipton Gentle Orange or Ginger Twist

What if you've forgotten to bring a bag of tea, and the restaurant has nothing good for the stomach? What can you do?

Go ahead and have some regular tea. But dip the teabag in the hot water for only about half a minute. If you do that, rather than let it steep, you'll end up getting about half as much caffeine. That quick-dip method also lowers the tannins, but you'll still get the tea flavor. Then, if you want to sweeten the tea a bit, you can add some skim milk or just one package (teaspoonful) of table sugar.

THE ABC'S OF McD'S

Yes, there are ways to get through McDonald's without incurring a lot of stomach distress. In fact, the method I recommend is as simple as A, B, C:

A. Order the apple oat bran muffin and skim or low-fat milk.

B. If you won't do A and you feel that you must have a sandwich, order an Egg McMuffin without the cheese, or throw away the bun half to which it clings.

C. Don't order the hash browns or the coffee.

SNACKING ON THE RUN

Snacking is fairly simple. Here are some foods to keep within reach:

➧ Whole wheat soft pretzels and mustard

➧ Yogurt, plain, plus a 1/2-ounce packet of jam (raspberry, strawberry, or orange marmalade)

➧ Lowest-sugar fruit yogurt you can find

➧ Hummus with pita wedges

➧ Grilled chicken salad, plain or with a sprinkle of oil and vinegar

➧ Baked corn chips with a non-spicy bean dip

➧ Baked potato with broccoli but no cheese

DINING OUT FOR LUNCH AND SUPPER

Recommended dishes:

➧ Chicken or chicken rice soup with oyster or saltine crackers

➧ Vegetable soup: bean, lentil, or pea (not tomato)

➧ Sandwich of smoked or roasted turkey breast or chicken breast (You can add some lowfat mozzarella or Swiss cheese. Serve on whole wheat or rye bread, garnished with lettuce and sprinkled with olive oil.)

➧ Garden Burger on whole wheat with lettuce

➧ Green salad with a sprinkle of olive oil and vinegar

➧ Grilled chicken salad

➧ Pasta salad with a sprinkle of oil and vinegar

➧ Broiled fish

➧ Chunk tuna(canned, packed in water) and green salad

➧ Roast chicken breast

Want some suggestions on what to avoid? Avoid tacos and burritos, because of their fat content and spice. Also, stay away from fried take-out Chinese food, since it's very high in fat. And don't try a tomato-sauce-laden pizza; all that acidic tomato sauce is too much for your stomach.

Got to have a burger? Order a small one with no cheese, onion, tomato, or ketchup. If you're getting a shake, ask for the low-fat version. As for fries, don't order them. This isn't a low-fat meal, but it's moderate fat and low acid, and it's less likely to give you rebound hyperacidity, heartburn, and esophageal reflux.

Hankering for Chinese? Order the Buddha's Delight—stir-fried vegetables, usually without garlic, with ginger root slices. Ask for peanuts on top to give the dish more protein. Ask for brown rice instead of white rice if they have it; it is absorbed more slowly and has more protein, vitamins, and minerals.

You'll do best with steamed dishes, but if they're not available, order a non-breaded chicken, pork, beef, or shrimp dish. Then ask for vegetables that are steamed instead of stir-fried.

Can't do without pizza? Order a small one and top it with ham and pineapple or broccoli and mushrooms, but no tomato sauce. (I suggest ham because it's lean and non-spicy, as opposed to sausage and, especially, pepperoni.)

The Subway chain features low-fat sandwiches. When you ask for oil, it's olive oil, and they don't use much of it.

Wendy's has a salad bar and will produce a low-fat, high-protein potato dish when it's requested. Just ask for a baker with cottage cheese and broccoli.

Wendy's, Burger King, and McDonald's all have grilled white-meat chicken, in a salad or a sandwich. The Have-It-Your-Way people will also provide a veggie sandwich when asked—all the salad greens you want in a bun.

The beverage lists at all of these places are not so good for dyspeptics. But you can always get water, which may be the only nonirritating choice.

A deli sandwich is fine if you choose lean meat, no cheese except Swiss or mozzarella (about 20% fat), and veggie greens. Hold the mayo, mustard, onions, and pickles.

Can you go to a nearby restaurant where they cook everything from scratch? It's the best way to control what goes into you. Try an Indian, Thai, or other Asian restaurant. If they attend to your needs well, think about becoming a regular at the place. Eating well-prepared food in a restaurant where your preferences are known is by far the best way to help your stomach, short of cooking everything for yourself.

Chapter 4

STRESS MANAGEMENT: DO YOU NEED IT?

In controlled trials, researchers found that many people who had chronic functional (non-ulcer) dyspepsia could be helped by psychotherapy treatments. This was true even when people were already getting medical treatments. In fact, in one study, all the patients had received two or more medical treatments during the previous six months, but those treatments alone did not resolve their problems.

What these studies tell us is that stomach and esophageal distress is not all in the esophagus and stomach. It's at least partly in the head. So, stress management is important to obtain lasting relief.

Most people who have non-ulcer dyspepsia are likely to have something else going on as well—anxiety, depression, hostility, tension, a history of childhood abuse, or plain old stress about garden-variety life events. Even ulcer patients are more prone to flare-ups of their illness if they feel stressed. So it's vital to develop ways to manage stress and the psychological problems that flow from it.

CAPSULE RECOMMENDATIONS ON STRESS MANAGEMENT

If you have stomach trouble, you probably have stress and need to learn to manage it. Then the big question is: Given all the choices of stress management that are offered, which is the most productive way for *you* to deal with stress?

For most of us, the better question is, what stress-control method will be rewarding enough, and easy enough, that we'll stick with it?

You can hardly tell what will work without trying options. You have to find something that clicks for you.

But still, what should you try first?

The broadest approach, and therefore the one most likely to work, is to take a **course in stress management**. These courses usually involve just a few hours of classroom work, along with some simple exercises that you do outside of the classroom.

The next most direct approach is **counseling**. If counseling focuses on identifying stresses and finding the means to cope with them, you can get lasting benefits after only a few sessions. Do not jump into it blindly, though. There are many approaches, and in my view, some are much more effective than others.

Psychodynamic-interpersonal therapy, a focused approach, has recently been proven more effective than supportive therapy even for functional dyspepsia in the toughest imaginable cases.

Group support is a worthwhile adjunct or sustainer if counseling has been helping. But you can't replace counseling if what you basically need is to learn how to deal with stress.

Relaxation training, **meditation**, and **prayer** are certainly worthwhile alternatives. But if your stomach problems are directly related to stress, you'll only get indirect benefits from these alternatives.

EXERCISE, THE STRESS RELIEVER

No matter how you tackle the mental, emotional, and spiritual aspects of stress reduction, you must, in addition, adopt a physical means of stress reduction. Exercise is vital! It's important to find a form of exercise that doesn't make you more tense or exhausted than you were before you started exercising. Do you feel exhilarated and relaxed when you've finished exercising? If not, I'd advise you to find another form of movement.

Whatever exercise you do for your body, it must help relax you afterward. If walking is too boring for you, or if your neighborhood isn't conducive to it, then dance. It takes hardly any space; it requires no partner; it only requires some music, legs that can move, and a heart that can handle more exercise than walking. Don't twist your back to the beat; step in time.

If you need deeper physical relaxation than you feel after your exercise, I recommend trying yoga first. (See more about this topic in

Chapter 6.) It is so instantly helpful that it has to be ranked number one among relaxing exercises.

If your body craves still more, try aerobics or kickboxing or some other guided exercise program—with monitoring by an expert coach—and stick with it for at least two weeks.

If you choose a guided exercise program, ease into it. Stand in the back of the class and don't try to keep up with the more experienced class members in the first week. Also, be sure to give your body a day off between classes. Otherwise, you will get too sore, and you might not persevere to the point where you begin to realize some benefits.

If all these means fail, or if you're quite certain that you need a skilled professional to get the benefit you need, try bodywork therapy. The specific type of therapy could be massage, chiropractic, or whatever appeals to you. But be sure that the therapy is done by a licensed professional.

$\mathcal{B}$ODYWORK THERAPY

Research has shown that therapeutic massage can reduce stress as well as exercise does. In osteopathic medicine, for instance, doctors use both regular medicine and therapeutic bodywork. Chiropractic is another form of bodywork therapy. A chiropractor aligns the body for an unimpeded flow of vital forces through the nervous system and peripheral nerves. Or you can simply have a massage. For the shy, an easy way to try this out is with a chair massage; that way you don't have to disrobe at all. It's soothing and relaxing.

Needless to say, you don't want to put pressure on the abdomen through forceful manipulation if you've been eating recently (say, within the past couple of hours). Apart from that caution, these systems can be a boon.

$\mathcal{I}$DENTIFYING STRESSES

How stressed are you? It might not even be necessary to ask that question, since so many people live with daily stress. How does your stress stack up against other people's? To find out, take the three Stress Measurement Tests that follow.

STRESS MEASUREMENT #1
How Do You Compare?

Here's a brief standard test that's used by many researchers to help determine stress levels.

As you read the questions below, think about the last month. Read the number key after each question, then write a number in each box, based on your first impulse. (You'll total the numbers when you're done.)

1. How often have you been upset because of something that happened unexpectedly?

   [__]   0 = never   1 = almost never   2 = sometimes
          3 = fairly often 4 = very often

2. How often have you felt that you were unable to control the important things in your life?

   [__]   0 = never   1 = almost never   2 = sometimes
          3 = fairly often 4 = very often

3. How often have you felt nervous and "stressed"?

   [__]   0 = never   1 = almost never   2 = sometimes
          3 = fairly often 4 = very often

4. How often have you felt confident about your ability to handle your personal problems?

   [__]   4 = never   3 = almost never   2 = sometimes
          1 = fairly often 0 = very often

5. How often have you felt that things were going your way?

   [__]   4 = never   3 = almost never   2 = sometimes
          1 = fairly often 0 = very often

6. How often have you been able to control irritations in your life?

   [__]   4 = never   3 = almost never   2 = sometimes
          1 = fairly often 0 = very often

7. How often have you found that you could not cope with all the things that you had to do?

   [__]   0 = never   1 = almost never   2 = sometimes
          3 = fairly often 4 = very often

8. How often have you felt that you were on top of things?

   [__]   4 = never   3 = almost never   2 = sometimes
            1 = fairly often   0 = very often

9. How often have you been angered because of things that were outside your control?

   [__]   0 = never   1 = almost never   2 = sometimes
            3 = fairly often   4 = very often

10. How often have you felt difficulties were piling up so high that you could not overcome them?

    [__]   0 = never   1 = almost never   2 = sometimes
             3 = fairly often   4 = very often

    [__]   YOUR TOTAL SCORE FOR ALL TEN ITEMS

Now you can compare your score against the average scores that were registered for various specific groups.

AVERAGE SCORES, BY SEX

Men	12.1
Women	13.7

AVERAGE SCORES, BY AGE

18–29	14.2
30–44	13.0
45–54	12.6
55–64	11.9
65 & over	12.0

AVERAGE SCORES, BY MARITAL STATUS

Widowed	12.6
Married or living with	12.4
Single or never wed	14.1
Divorced	14.7
Separated	16.6

Is your score above or below the average for the group you're in? If it's below, then perhaps you should consider that stress is not a very big problem for you. Other factors may be playing a much bigger role in causing or contributing to gastrointestinal problems. If you're below average on all three demographic groupings, it seems you have little to fret about.

On the other hand, if your scores are significantly higher than average, you may need to give attention to compensating with specific strategies that are designed to bring you relief. Major stresses have long-lasting after-effects. You'll probably have to focus on these chronic stresses if you hope to succeed in dealing with stomach illness.

STRESS MEASUREMENT TEST 2
Causes of Long-Term Stress

This survey is a comprehensive overview of the many possible causes of long-term stress. It's called the Recent Experience Scale, and it was compiled by Thomas H. Holmes, M.D., at the Department of Psychiatry and Behavioral Sciences, University of Washington School of Medicine.

When you're considering your answers to the first part of this survey, think about what's happened during the past year. Turning to the second part, think about things that have happened to you during the past *two* years.

RECENT EXPERIENCE SCALE

Part 1. Think back on each possible life event listed below. Decide if it happened to you within the last year. If the event did happen, use the score that's shown. If the event didn't happen, just leave the line blank immediately after the number.

RECENT EXPERIENCE (IN PRIOR YEAR)	SCORE
1. A lot more or a lot less trouble with boss	23 ____
2. A major change in sleeping habits (sleeping a lot more or a lot less, or a change in the part of the day when you've been sleeping)	16 ____
3. A major change in eating habits (a lot more or a lot less food intake, different meal hours or surroundings)	15 ____

RECENT EXPERIENCE (IN PRIOR YEAR)	SCORE	
4. A revision of personal habits (dress, manners, associations etc.)	24	___
5. A major change in usual type and/or amount of recreation	19	___
6. A major change in social activities (a lot more or a lot less than usual)	18	___
7. A major change in religious group activities (a lot more or a lot less than usual)	19	___
8. A major change in number of family get-togethers (a lot more or a lot fewer than usual)	15	___
9. A major change in financial state (a lot worse off or a lot better off than previously)	38	___
10. In-law troubles	29	___
11. A major change in number of arguments with spouse regarding child-rearing, personal habits, and other issues (a lot more or a lot fewer than usual)	35	___
12. Sexual difficulties	39	___

Part 2. In the space provided, indicate the number of times that each event happened to you within the last **two** years. Then multiply that number by the score that's provided to get a total score for each type of experience.

EXPERIENCE	NUMBER OF TIMES	MEAN VALUE	SCORE
13. Major personal injury or illness	___	53	___
14. Death of spouse	___	100	___
15. Death of close family member (not spouse)	___	63	___
16. Death of a close friend	___	37	___
17. Gaining new family member (birth, aged parent moving in, adoption, etc.)	___	39	___

EXPERIENCE	TIMES	VALUE	SCORE
18. Major change in health or behavior of family member	____	44	____
19. Change in residence	____	20	____
20. Detention in jail or other institution	____	63	____
21. Major business readjustment (merger, reorganization, bankruptcy, etc.)	____	39	____
22. Minor violations of the law	____	11	____
23. Marriage	____	50	____
24. Divorce	____	73	____
25. Marital separation	____	65	____
26. Outstanding personal achievement	____	28	____
27. Son or daughter leaving home	____	29	____
28. Major change in working hours or conditions	____	20	____
29. Major change in responsibilities at work (promotion, demotion, transfer)	____	29	____
30. Retirement from work	____	45	____
31. Being fired or laid off from work	____	47	____
32. Major change in living conditions (new home, remodeling, deterioration, etc.)	____	25	____
33. Spouse beginning or ceasing work outside the home	____	26	____
34. Taking on mortgage greater than $100,000	____	31	____
35. Taking on mortgage less than $100,000	____	17	____
36. Foreclosure on mortgage or loan	____	30	____
37. Vacation	____	13	____
38. Changing to a new school	____	20	____

EXPERIENCE	TIMES	VALUE	SCORE
39. Changing to a different line of work	____	36	____
40. Beginning or ceasing formal schooling	____	26	____
41. Marital reconciliation	____	45	____
42. Pregnancy	____	40	____
43. Christmas	____	12	____

TOTAL ____

INTERPRETING YOUR SCORE

A score of 300 or more gives you an 80% likelihood of developing a major illness in the near future. Let's hope your score isn't that high. If it is, there are many things you can do to de-stress.

STRESS MEASUREMENT TEST 3
What's Your Response to Stress?

Apart from specific experiences that might be causing stress, most of us habitually respond to stress in certain ways. That is, some people have stress-prone personalities, and some people roll with the punches. Here's a brief survey to help you determine whether you have a stress-prone personality.

STRESS-PRONE PERSONALITY

	ALMOST NEVER (5)	RARELY (4)	SOME-TIMES (3)	OFTEN (2)	ALMOST ALWAYS (1)
1. Talk loud and fast					
2. Remember facts and figures					
3. Am annoyed when I have to wait					
4. Take on more than I should					
5. Work hard; go at "full speed"					
6. Feel resentment about things					
7. Become angry enough to hit or throw things					
8. Am irritated by inefficiency					

STRESS-PRONE PERSONALITY *(cont'd)*

	ALMOST NEVER (1)	RARELY (2)	SOME-TIMES (3)	OFTEN (4)	ALMOST ALWAYS (5)
9. React to problems in an easy-going manner					
10. Listen well; don't interrupt others					
11. Have/make time for relaxation					
12. Work at an unhurried, steady pace					
13. Spend time in leisure pursuits; take a walk, read, etc.					
14. Make decisions slowly and deliberately					
15. Avoid being the one to run things					
16. Am satisfied with present position and status					
Subtotals of each column					

TOTAL SCORE _____

Interpret the degree to which you are prone to the adverse effects of stress as follows:

16–33   Type A: Highly vulnerable to adverse effects of stress.

45–59   Type AB: May be vulnerable to adverse effects of stress in some situations.

60–80   Type B: Not very vulnerable to adverse effects of stress at this time.

Chapter 5

STRESS MANAGEMENT STRATEGIES

One of the best ways to learn stress management strategies is by taking a course that helps you deal with stressful situations. Usually, the course helps students by outlining many possible avenues of help. A course can start you thinking about how to help yourself in many different situations. For instance:

➠ Avoid hassles. Take time to develop strategies for this. If rush-hour traffic bothers you, find out if you can use flextime to drive to and from work earlier or later than rush hour. Or try car-pooling or using public transportation.

➠ If you're snappish with your spouse when you are hungry, start stocking your pantry or fridge with healthy snacks and march yourself to the kitchen to eat one when you need to. If your main fights begin late at night, get yourself to bed early. Your peace of mind is more precious than another hour of entertainment by television in the late evening, isn't it?

➠ Control the number of changes that hit you all at once. When any change, good or bad, happens, deliberately keep up with the other activities that you enjoy.

➠ Take a break. When you feel you can't cope, go to the water cooler or the rest room for a minute. Stretch your legs. If you can't get away from it all, at least stretch out and take a deep breath. Take a few seconds to mentally rearrange your priorities for the next hour or more.

➦ Find help when the out-of-control or can't-catch-up feeling persists. Your employer may have an Employee Assistance Plan (EAP) with counselors available on very short notice. They help—and there may be no charge at all for the first several sessions.

$\mathcal{C}$OUNSELING

Maybe you've been to doctor after doctor, followed their instructions religiously, and still you have stomach trouble.

What if you go to your doctor thinking you have a legitimate medical problem with your stomach, and he or she advises a counseling program? Hold up before you retort, angrily, that the problem is *not* all in your head.

Seeking counseling is not a sign of weakness or craziness. It is not giving someone else license to "play with" your head. It is sound, scientifically proven treatment for real problems. Nowadays, counseling is often a specific, focused program comprised of about a dozen sessions (and many health plans don't pay for more than that).

There are many kinds of therapists and counselors. Some say no one has a mental disorder, that everyone is unique and has his or her own combination of problems and own truth. This is very respectful and even poetic, but it may not give you any quick help with your stomach.

If you do go for counseling, it's very unlikely that the therapist will invite you to lie back on a couch and engage in a totally undirected flow of associations and memories. That Freudian stuff is still practiced by a small fraction of therapists, but it's a years-long approach to a problem that needs faster relief.

Most therapists will ask directed questions and thus get a reasonably good idea in just an hour or two of what ails you. That doesn't mean a therapist can instantly decide what's wrong with your stomach; but he or she can help you identify your "erroneous zones"—that is, how you mistreat yourself and how you act with and react to others.

Just because therapists ask directed questions, however, that doesn't mean they make snap judgments. Nor does it mean that they are omniscient seers who can read you like a book. No one can learn everything relevant about you in an hour. But it should only take a session or two to establish goals and a treatment plan with you.

Several therapy systems have now shown solid proof of medical efficacy for specific conditions such as depression, a particularly common illness with a great deal of bodily symptoms, particularly of the GI tract.

Depending on who you see, your therapist may concentrate on how to relate realistically and productively to the other people who are important to you. This is known as **interpersonal therapy**. Others will train you out of self-defeating behaviors and into self-affirming, successful behaviors; that's the process of **behavior therapy** or behavior modification. Still others will help you change how you perceive yourself and the world, helping you to blossom from a healthier inner perspective; that's **cognitive therapy**.

Each of the many systems can do no more than polish a facet of the whole mind, but each lets the light in. Some therapists call themselves "eclectic" because they know how to work in more than one system and, hence, treat more than one facet of the mind.

What's the best of all therapy systems? In my view, the best therapist is the one who helps you most. Just as a particular physician may not suit every patient because of his or her manner, not every competent counselor or therapist is right for every client. So, before you take the plunge into counseling, interview a therapist or two for a few minutes.

$\mathcal{B}$EFORE YOU START WITH A THERAPIST

Good therapists will give you forthright information about themselves, and they'll be happy to answer the questions you ask. Ask about their training and license. Ask what kind of treatment they believe in and practice. Ask how many patients with your kind of problems they have counseled. Remember: You are auditioning them, not vice versa.

The process of interviewing a therapist helps break the ice and establish a working relationship. It gets you started on a partner-like basis. You're not prostrating yourself or becoming a dependent. The partnership begins with the interview.

After you start out, don't be afraid to request a review periodically. "What would you say have been my main problems among what I've told you? Where are we going? What are your goals for me? Have they changed recently?"

Also, review for yourself periodically:

➠ *Do I like and respect this counselor?* At least one "yes" is a must.

➠ *Does she challenge me, or just reassure me?* You don't need to hear "You'll be fine" like a broken record. If that were so, why come to therapy?

➠ *If he provokes or annoys me, do I eventually see a worthwhile result from it?* Getting angry at the counselor is not necessarily bad. You may need someone to get mad at, and therapists are tough. They know that the real target is usually somebody else and that you don't want to face it, or show it. That's part of why your stomach is churning.

➠ *Do I feel that we're making progress?* You may well feel stuck for a few weeks. But if there's never any feeling of breakthrough, don't blame it all on either party, but also don't just keep shelling out your money and your time. Find a more dynamic counselor.

➠ *Is she taking control of me?* This causes backsliding into greater mental problems unless you're almost certifiably, totally out of control.

➠ *Is he helping me to find options for myself?* This is excellent if the client wants to be an adult.

ℛESEARCH SUPPORT

Specific forms of psychotherapy have been proven effective for treating dyspepsia. A 1994 study proved that cognitive therapy, a short-term form of psychotherapy that has been proven effective for treatment of depression and anxiety (also called cognitive behavior therapy), was more effective to relieve functional dyspepsia than routine treatment by gastroenterologists. For the best-proven specific type of therapy, ask for psychodynamic-interpersonal (PI) therapy, which was developed in Britain.

PI therapy beat supportive therapy in the study results. Although PI therapy is not yet widely available in the United States, it's very similar to Interpersonal Therapy (IPT), which *is* easily available in the U.S.

PI emphasizes the formation of a strong collaboration, a working alliance, between therapist and patient for exploring, revealing, and modifying the patient's interpersonal difficulties. Best of all, it shows benefits after just seven sessions. Since IPT is similar, you might get equally good results.

*G*ROUP SUPPORT

Gastroenterology has not been blessed with a great popularizer of group support or general mind-body medicine. Cardiology has Dr. Dean Ornish, though, and the field of chronic pain treatment has Jon Kabat-Zinn. These two mind-body healers have helped legions conquer their diseases and their pain. They both recommend exercise, relaxation, yoga, and meditation. But they both say that is not enough. What provides a new kind of relief and the sustaining motivation to continue the work of the program, they have found, is group support and sharing.

Dr. Ornish uses the term "opening your heart" very deliberately to describe his program. He brings together small groups of his patients and strongly encourages them to tell each other how they are feeling and what led them to join the program. Soon they find that, no matter how diverse their backgrounds and education, they have something in common. It's not just their heart disease; it's their basic humanity. Paradoxically, by opening their hearts, they take heart.

Kabat-Zinn teaches much the same thing to his chronic pain patients. No matter how severe the pain, it lessens at least a little when shared. The dam of holding feelings inside also holds illness in.

You probably won't have to look very far to find a support group. You'll see notices in health food stores, or you can ask through your doctor, check at your local hospital, or phone a mental health agency. Most professional counselors facilitate (not "run") support groups for a small fee. The phone company's Infoline and Twelve-Step hotlines in your area make referrals, too.

If you are confused about what support group to try for stress management, because you don't have any addiction except to Rolaids, you might start with Codependents Anonymous. The vast majority of us seem to be plagued with this insidious virus—98 percent of us, according to Barry and Janae Weinhold, authors of one self-help text on the subject.

Precautions about support groups:

➡ *They're not a substitute for professional counseling.* If going to the group sessions doesn't help or at least comfort you after two or three sessions, ask for professional, individual help.

➡ *You may feel out of place the first time you attend a group.* You may want to run out before the hour is up. That's not a bad sign; that usually means it's hitting you where you hurt. Hang in there, and face the music. Listen with respect rather than judgment to the tribulations that the speakers are baring. The fact that they attend and bear witness to their issues demonstrates their desire to change for the better. Say a little about yourself to at least one person.

➡ *If there is a facilitator, note how open he or she is to the natural bonding that flows from shared problems and interests.* Beware the facilitator who forbids lunching or other joint activities by smaller groups or pairs of the participants. That may be important for a therapy group, where everybody's got to stay in the know about each other's problems, and working things out all together is crucial. But it's inappropriate for support groups.

➡ *Beware the facilitator who holds a position of authority and doesn't admit his or her own humanity.* You are trying to learn how to manage your own life; it does you no good in the long run if an authority makes decisions for you or tells you what to do. The most arrogant such individuals are those who won't acknowledge their own failures, weaknesses, distresses, or unsolved problems.

➡ *Determine how comfortable you are with the rules of the house.* Some groups forbid talking about others, especially those who are present. That can be great for keeping good boundaries in the group (not to mention avoiding fights), but it may seem too cold to you. Most groups forbid interrupting others as they speak and until they say they are finished talking. That can frustrate your urges to "help," but learning to let people walk their own paths may be an important lesson for you. You can always wait until the end of the meeting and then approach someone whose remarks particularly struck you.

Chapter 6

DISPELLING YOUR STRESS WITH RELAXATION, YOGA, MEDITATION, AND PRAYER

In many groups you'll learn stress management techniques that you can use on your own. These include relaxation, meditation, prayer, and yoga.

Dr. Herbert Benson at Harvard University has researched the physiological changes that follow a simple form of relaxing for ten or twenty minutes while concentrating on a positive word or phrase. The Relaxation Response that follows includes lower pulse and blood pressure, slower breathing, and a change in the brain-wave pattern to slower cycles called alpha waves.

The word or phrase can be the briefest of affirmations, such as "peace," or a prayer, such as "love to all." The response occurs within minutes and continues for hours. Practicing this technique twice a day is recommended for full effects.

Drs. Jon Kabat-Zinn and Saki Santorelli at the University of Massachusetts Center for Mindfulness in Medicine, Health Care, and Society (Worcester, MA) have rescued sufferers of intractable chronic pain from 90 percent of their symptoms. The doctors coached the patients, helping them practice a technique similar to the relaxation response called Mindfulness Meditation.

Kabat-Zinn and Santorelli tried two other methods as well. They asked patients to share their issues with a supportive group. They also had patients practice stretching exercises—the equivalent of hatha yoga.

WRITE IT UP

In a controlled study, other researchers found that people who write about their problems and struggles for a few minutes each day can increase their immune function significantly. Since decreased immune function is a direct result of stress, an increase in immune function could easily be a good index of decreased stress. In the study, the key to success was steering the writing away from a nonemotional recitation of the day's events in favor of venting about problems. Apparently this "closet psychotherapy" led to resolution of problems, at least among the volunteers. And it took only three days!

Stress management courses often include relaxation training. One popular method is called deep muscle relaxation or progressive relaxation. Using this technique, people learn about relaxation by practicing its opposite, tension.

PROGRESSIVE RELAXATION

To begin progressive relaxation, first lie down comfortably on your back. Breathe in slowly and, while you do, tighten all the muscles in one leg, pitting them against one another. Strain the muscles tighter and tighter for a couple of seconds while you lift your leg about an inch above the floor.

⇒ With a big sigh, let the leg fall. Move it from side to side a couple of times, then relax it.

⇒ Do the same with the other leg.

⇒ Then do the tensing and relaxing exercise with your buttocks.

⇒ Progress to the abdomen, pushing it out with a big in-breath.

⇒ Then move to the chest: Take a big in-breath, then release.

⇒ Strain one arm, then the other.

⇒ Tense the muscles around your head and neck. Squinching your eyes and mouth shut, raise your head an inch before letting it fall with a sigh.

➡ Open your eyes and mouth as wide as you can and stick out your tongue, then relax with a sigh.

➡ Finally, lie back and enjoy the feeling of complete relaxation. If any tension remains, go through the sequence again.

OTHER RELAXATION APPROACHES

There must be a million other ways of concentrating the mind to achieve a relaxed state. Luxuriate in a sauna or a hot bath. Use sound: Play an instrument, sing, chant, drum, or learn how to make a Tibetan bowl sing. Isn't it amazing how great, dedicated musicians often live to a ripe old age? There's a lesson there about stress.

YOGA CLASSES

There are many kinds of yoga, some quite arcane and religious. But one, hatha yoga, is recommended over and over again because it gives you health benefits without forcing you to follow any particular philosophy or subscribe to a certain theology. For hatha yoga, you don't need to be at any particular fitness level to get started. And you don't have to tie yourself into pretzels, adopting the famous yoga positions that intimidate so many people.

Hatha yoga is mostly just stretches, but in time-honored positions and patterns that aid the body. Breathing exercises are an integral part of the practice, and so is a relaxation exercise and a meditation at the end of each session.

The most unusual thing you might have to do is to chant a few phrases that set a tone (literally) for the class, but that is practiced in a small minority of the yoga classes that I've attended.

It's best to learn hatha yoga from an instructor. That's the surest way to avoid developing bad habits that cause pain, strain, or worse. If you don't know where to start or whom to ask, try your YMCA. Yes, hatha yoga is so mainstream that it's taught at the Y!

Will the instructor be expert enough to meet your needs? There's only one way to find out: Try it. If the instructor starts with music, you're in the wrong hands. If there's quiet in the room, and if the instructor makes you feel at ease, you're off to a promising start.

If the instructor demonstrates each pose, watches you and helps guide you in doing it, supports one and all in a relaxed way, and gives each of you a chance to catch your breath before the next pose, you're on your way. After the first class, if you feel relaxed, refreshed, even mildly high, you're definitely in the right place.

If not—if you feel tired, stressed, or overwhelmed by your failure to keep up with the class—look around for another instructor.

$\mathcal{Y}$OGA VIDEOS

Too shy to start in a group? There are excellent yoga videotapes available. Just don't be put off by the demonstrations at the beginning. They always seem to feature an impossibly slim and lithe instructor.

Good form does not count in yoga! All that matters is following the instruction to the point of feeling a good stretch, and not hurting oneself by straining. I particularly recommend the series of videotapes produced by *Yoga Journal*, especially the one called "Yoga For Flexibility."

$\mathcal{G}$OING BY THE BOOKS

Are you someone who likes to assimilate new material more slowly? Do you want to flip some pages in a book about yoga before you consider flipping yourself about on the floor? Try the chapter on yoga in *Dr. Dean Ornish's Program for Reversing Heart Disease*. The instruction in hatha yoga is excellent, and the picture sequences are unusually easy to understand.

A somewhat more ambitious read but still very easy to understand is *Yoga the Iyengar Way* by Silva, Mira, and Shyam Mehta. The foreword in it, and the methods it espouses, are by B.K.S. Iyengar, the modern master who popularized yoga in the West. Iyengar accomplished this in part by bringing the comforting expedients of props and cushions into the practice.

Yoga the Iyengar Way is chock-full of color pictures of yogis performing the asanas (pronounced AH-san-nas). A great consolation in it is seeing that about half of the models are pleasantly plump rather than willowy or emaciated.

$\mathcal{T}$RY IT!

Here's the classic asana, one to use at the end of every workout whether you've been doing yoga or exercising in some other way. Lie down on your back on a firm but not hard surface—a carpet is fine, or a cushion on the floor. If the small of your back or your neck does not like this, take up the empty space by inserting a rolled-up towel. Cover up with enough clothes or a blanket so that you won't get chilled from lying still.

Get comfortable. Spread your legs so your feet lie about a foot apart and let the toes splay, relaxed. Spread your arms a few inches from your body and let the palms roll up comfortably.

Breathe through your nose. Pay attention as you breathe. Notice how cool your nostrils feel as each breath enters. Notice the warmth as you expel each breath. Pay attention to your chest, how it rises and falls with each breath. Pay attention to your whole body, lying relaxed. Let it sink or float as it may, a little more with the extra relaxation of each exhalation.

Don't think, don't count the breaths, don't do anything but breathe, relax, and concentrate on the breathing.

This is called *pose of the dead* or *corpse pose, savasana* in Sanskrit. The name is a sly attempt to get students to emulate the ultimate form of total relaxation, not to get them spooked. A few minutes of savasana is highly refreshing. Or, if you are overtired, it may put you to sleep.

When you feel ready to resume activities, take a few deeper breaths, wriggle your toes and fingers, stretch, and flutter your eyes open slowly. Rise slowly and gently by rolling onto your right side and pushing up with both arms.

$\mathcal{D}$ISCIPLINE AND FREEDOM

The practice of yoga goes from as little oxygen consumption as in savasana up to the grueling super-workout called ashtanga yoga. You can take it as far as you like.

Ten minutes a day in well-directed poses may be all you need to calm your stomach and all of the rest of you. Half an hour at the beginning of the day is likely to relax you for the whole morning's work.

Paradoxically, ten to thirty minutes of asanas can provide a refreshing way to start an evening that gives you zest for activities or a partner.

The practice of yoga helps you achieve discipline and freedom. I don't mean discipline as in punishment, but discipline as in making your body and spirit your disciples.

How can yoga help you achieve freedom if it leads you to discipline yourself? By giving you a practiced will, confidence that you can withstand discomfort and go the distance to reach goals. This is the real requirement for a free life.

Yet all of these benefits are not the ultimate goal of yoga. That is becoming one with your deepest self—God, if you believe—usually through service and altruism.

THE POWER OF MEDITATION

Meditation is incredibly simple yet incredibly deep. It is so accessible to the novice that it's a great compliment to experienced practitioners to achieve "beginner's mind." This is the delight in savoring what is new about it. And yet there is no end to all of the rich "places" inside where meditation can lead.

Serenity, refreshment, and relaxation are early attainments. Finding more meaning in life and an interior spirituality soon come also. Meditation has been described as a voyage to an infinite internal world and as an opening to the guidance of the greatest teacher.

It takes only a minute to try it. I recall instant disappointment at discovering that there's really nothing to it when I first started reading the American bible on the practice, *Be Here Now*, by Ram Dass. My reaction was, "Is that all it is? I don't feel a thing."

Ram Dass is a Harvard biological researcher (his original name was Richard Alpert) who had worked with Timothy Leary on the early human experiments with LSD. He became disenchanted with the limitation of achieving spiritual communion only through a chemical, so he went to India to find a guru. Following the teachings of his guru, Alpert changed his name to Ram Dass and renounced his scientific skepticism. The apprentice worked to spread the power his teacher invoked—meditation—throughout the Western world.

𝒮UNDAMENTALS OF MEDITATION

All meditation requires is being still (sitting, standing, or lying) in a comfortable position in a quiet place, and concentrating on something so simple that the mind can no longer be described as "thinking."

Ways to do this can be anything from saying "peace" again and again, to concentrating on the breath going in and out of the body from the nose to the lungs and back. Or you can concentrate on other of the body's signals, even discomforts.

It is only by trying this that one discovers what a chatterbox the mind is. Within seconds of starting a meditation (unless you fall asleep), you will start remembering chores you've forgotten to do, or a phone message you need to answer, or maybe a pop song that plays endlessly inside your head.

You'll get a brilliant idea you feel you must write down immediately before you lose it forever. Or you'll think of a new strategy to deal with someone who's been annoying you. It's amazing—but it's not meditation.

Meditation calls for gently, passively bringing the mind back to your plan—the breath, the word or phrase, the mindful attention to the body—whatever you intended as your method to meditate.

𝒟EALING WITH DISTRACTION

Wayne Dyer, author of *Your Erroneous Zones* and *Meditations for Manifesting*, recommends transcendental meditation. TM, as it's called, is so popular that you can probably find a local trainer in the Yellow Pages.

In one of Dyer's audiotape series, he talks about how he got up at dawn to meditate at a beautiful resort in Hawaii. This highly experienced meditator, a man of serenity and peace, experienced such distraction that he quickly became enraged, close to the point of committing violence. The source of the distraction happened to be external. A groundskeeper was operating one of those gas-powered edgers, not the little kind with the whippy string but the kind that grind the grass away from the sidewalk like a demented aircraft engine, one of those insanely noisy machines. Dr. Dyer kept his eyes closed, but the din seemed so close, so quadraphonically enveloping, that he thought the groundsman must have been edging the very blanket on which Dyer was meditating.

Dr. Dyer probably saved himself from injury (and, quite likely, an assault charge) by remembering one of his own teachings. The author said he realized that, whatever is going on, he always had a choice in how he would respond. Soon he forgave the interruption and reached an even deeper level of meditation than usual.

This is what it takes to deal with distraction: forgiving yourself for being distracted, and forgiving the distraction. Thank your mind for reminding you about that chore; it's only trying to help. Bless your brain for thinking up a way to deal with that person who's bugging you. The old bean has been taking care of your schedule for a lot of years. You don't want to lay it off or fire it. You just want to give it a rest for a few minutes.

And yet you still may only be able to do so for about five seconds at a time. I recall taking a class in professional-level meditation. After the class was over, I sheepishly admitted to two other members of the class that I couldn't really meditate for more than about five seconds. Since I expected to be ridiculed, their enthusiastic support came as a complete surprise. They both exclaimed, "That's good! Five seconds is a great start!"

Don't worry; the time spent in the state of meditation becomes fruitful, no matter how variable the little bursts of letting go are.

$\mathcal{M}$INDFULNESS MEDITATION

Jack Kornfield and Jon Kabat-Zinn are famous for teaching Mindfulness Meditation. In this practice, you actually recruit some of the bodily distractions so they become part of the essence of meditation.

Mindfulness Meditation involves not only focusing on the breath but also focusing on the body in various ways. For instance, you do a "body scan," getting mentally in touch with how every part of your body feels, one small area at a time, progressing up from your toes. Before moving on to a new part, the sole of the foot for example, you breathe in and imagine the breath sending good things all the way to the toes. Then you breathe out, imagining the body part purified.

You don't even have to be still to do this. You can be on a treadmill or a ski machine or doing anything (safely) repetitious. I've been amazed how quickly and easily an aerobic workout goes when I meditate into a body scan as soon as I've accelerated through the warm-up phase of all that stepping.

Sufis meditate by whirling about, dancing. Drummers meditate by repeating their strokes, beating out the rhythm in a mesmerizing continuum of sound. Even eating or chewing gum can be a form of meditation.

Kabat-Zinn likes to lead into mindfulness by having a new class hold a single raisin awhile, smell it, put it on the tongue, and slowly chew it. A morsel for mindfulness.

READINGS TO START WITH

You can also start into meditation without trying to let go into non-thinking or into concentrating exclusively on a simple activity. There are some wonderful little books that artfully take the reader into a brief contemplation.

The Hazelden Meditation Series is based on the Twelve Steps, but it is not preachy. It includes a rich little starter book for men, *Touchstones*, and another for women, *Each Day a New Beginning*. Both have an entry for each day of the year. The little page (the books are palm-size) can be read in a minute or two, even reading slowly to savor the thought.

Of course, any of these books can be reread if you want to get into a little more depth. Or you can set the book aside and simply think about the day's reading for some minutes. Or perhaps you'd prefer to respond to the day's thought in a diary entry.

PRAYER, TOO

And then there's prayer. Dr. Benson of Harvard, the advocate of the Relaxation Response, endorses prayer, both for its immediate benefits and for the long-term rewards. Scientific studies show that belief in the divine can dramatically lower your risk of many kinds of illness.

Free-form prayer may seem more sincere to you, but rote prayer is also excellent for inducing the relaxation state.

TAKE A MIND TRIP

One way to meditate without blanking your mind out entirely is what I call trip meditation.

Get still in a comfortable position. Close your eyes. "Do" (imagine) a lead-in ritual. For instance, you might imagine walking up a staircase into a special room. Or count down through a small number of quiet breaths, perhaps ten of them.

Then imagine a favorite place where you have been. You are there again, alone and serene with being alone. Imagine what you see as yourself looking about, slowly. Imagine the sounds, perhaps of birds or insects or waves. Feel the wind. Imagine the smells on the air. Just don't name them or talk to yourself about them. Simply experience all the imagined sensations.

I have a trip meditation that I love. It starts with feeling cool, moist sand on my bare feet as I mosey along a deserted stretch of the Lake Michigan shore—the Long Blue Edge of Summer (in the felicitous phrase of one travel writer). Seagulls call, dip in the air, feed, strut the beach. I leave the lapping waves and plod slowly up a small dune.

At the rounded crest of the dune, I see ahead into a blowout, a wind-scooped valley one rise away from the big lake. I ease down the slope and sit my imaginary self down under a little pine. It sighs in the breeze. I gaze at a blue pond of rainwater along the far edge of the blowout. Its surface sparkles in the midday sun. I feel the sun heat my skin. The horizon, a series of low dunes spiked with pines and poplars, softened with swirls of long grasses, is comfortably near.

The seagull chorus is distant, soft in the background. The little valley enfolds me in peace.

■

What if you feel you haven't got an imagination, but you want to see something to concentrate on? Open a travel magazine and stare at a lovely scene. Then close your eyes, even for a few seconds, and imagine something about that scene. It's okay to peek if you need to. Practice will expand your ability to imagine.

Or just close your eyes and see what patterns your eyeballs or brain produce. Sometimes they are quite lovely and colorful. They dissolve and re-form or change from second to second, always renewing themselves. It's your internal screensaver.

When you've meditated as long as you care to, gently take a deep breath, wiggle your fingers and toes a little, stretch a bit, and slowly open your eyes.

When you rise, you may feel as if you're floating on a cloud for a while, that you are full of delight in people and impervious to all of the stress of life. It may not last for long, but if you do this kind of thing for ten or fifteen minutes a couple of times a day, you will do wonders for your body and soul.

For the practice of meditation, set aside a certain amount of time each day, or at least most days of the week. I know that may not sound easy. Time is a precious commodity. For most of us, it's in short supply. But consider your need, your hunger to feel better and find more in life. Doesn't that motivate you to try, and try again?

Part 2

APPLYING NUTRITIONAL PRINCIPLES

Chapter 7

$\mathcal{F}$IND
THE RIGHT CARBS

$\mathcal{W}$hen you digest carbohydrate, it turns into nothing but sugar—a substance that is often demonized by people who say it's terrible for us.

Yet, other people praise high-carbohydrate foods as the ones that will keep us from getting fat and will power us through anything, even a marathon. What's going on?

This is organic chemistry and biochemistry. Let's demystify it.

The organic compounds we call sugars are simple molecules that need little or no digestion before getting absorbed. With only half a dozen carbon atoms per molecule, they're tiny. Each molecule can slide right through the lining of the stomach and intestine and zoom into the bloodstream. So they're speedily absorbed, and that means, potentially, they're toxic fat-formers.

The sugars in starchy foods like cereals, pasta, potatoes, and rice are in the form of complex carbohydrates. A molecule of starch may have a million carbon atoms. It's a natural polymer, nature's own poly-glucose fiber.

Starch molecules are long strings of simple sugars chemically locked together in chains that are as tightly joined as the fibers in a piece of cotton. In fact, cotton fibers *are* poly-glucose. But the glucoses in starch aren't joined together the way they are in cotton. The ones in starch have a different twist.

Our digestive enzymes can't break down the complex carbohydrates in cotton. Saliva, however, is enough to digest starch. It has an enzyme, ptyalin, that breaks the links between glucose molecules in starch. So, good old saliva is actually a sophisticated biochemical processing agent. Another one, amylase from the pancreas, finishes the job in the small intestine.

♂OO MUCH SUGAR

Table sugar is also a carbohydrate, but it's the simple kind. Where I grew up in the Midwest, we called sweetened, carbonated beverages "pop." Not soda, as they say on the east coast. That word—pop!—actually said a lot about what we were drinking. The sugar in those drinks is enough to make some of us pop the buttons of our pants.

You know how a couple of teaspoons of sugar can make a cup of coffee or a glass of iced tea revoltingly sweet? Cola, lemon-lime, and similar carbonated beverages have about *six* teaspoons of sugar per cup, 90 calories worth. The other day, I saw an Arizona beverage label that showed the can contained 300 calories worth of sugars. A Big Gulp has over 500. That's over a cup of sugar, about a quarter of the total calorie requirements for an entire day for an adult.

One sugar company used to advertise that sugar was only 15 calories per teaspoon, and it was "all energy." This slogan is no longer used, because it is a lie. Sugar is used only for energy, not for making fat, if we eat no more food than we need, and if it is absorbed slowly. Otherwise, eating sugar makes us gain fat.

How did we get so hooked on sweet tastes? Well, sugar does have a pleasant taste, so it's more interesting than water. It's also cheap. And it's stable when acidified with carbon dioxide or pasteurized in fruit-flavored drinks.

But sugar is habit-forming; it produces *tolerance*. That is, gradually, you need to keep eating more sugar to get the same sensations of sweetness that you used to get with less.

If you don't believe this of sugar, try sucking on a hard candy and notice how boring it gets unless you work it around in your mouth or munch on it to keep increasing the concentration of sugar in your mouth. So, sugar answers the dreams of the food-making corporations: The more we eat, the more we need.

As I mentioned before, starch is nothing but sugar. But if that's true, why, then, does it have no sweet taste?

With molecules so huge, starch doesn't really dissolve. Instead, starch gets suspended in little particles in water. Yet, taste buds only work on solutions. With so few molecules per spoonful, starch hasn't much luck at tickling your taste buds.

Here's an example to prove how little taste you find in complex carbohydrates. Try a dash of cornstarch, plain. It's not much different from eating plain white bread. With so little flavor to tempt the taste buds, we generally go for the simple sugars and simple-sugar products (which are so sweet to the taste), and often ignore the starches because they don't have much flavor.

Starch does come in some pleasant-tasting, impure forms. You can get natural mixtures made of whole-grain cereals, potatoes, corn, and rice with the hull left on. Counting pasta, starch includes all the dietary staples that give the best combination of enough energy but slow digestion and absorption. Far better than simple sugars, these foods stay in the stomach longer and then stay in the intestine longer.

Staying in the stomach longer means they, and the juice with them, buffer stomach acid longer between meals. This means less *acid rebound* in the stomach.

Think of the last time you had a sugary breakfast without whole-grain cereal. Suppose, for instance, you had a donut and coffee. If you have GERD, or chronic indigestion, you may remember feeling bloated afterward, along with some belching. You're likely to have had a very uncomfortable feeling about 45 minutes or an hour after you finished your donut and coffee.

That discomfort is not something new and unrelated. Rather, it's acid rebound. Assaulted by the coffee and donut combination, your stomach starts churning out acid. Though food passes through the stomach fairly quickly, heavy acid flow is likely to continue a while. Soon, your stomach-acid tachometer is redlined.

If, instead, you eat food that digests slowly, you'll help to prevent the acid flow. Also, that slow-to-digest food makes another good thing happen in your stomach: If food stays in your stomach longer, you don't feel hungry as soon. So you'll be less apt to chase hunger pains by eating high-sugar snacks between meals.

Let's look at the way sugars and starches help cause a rise in blood sugar. From what I've already said, it may seem that I consider sugar the bad guy. Isn't it sugar (in food) that makes your blood sugar soar and then crash? Aren't starches the slow, sustaining heroes of blood sugar?

It's not so simple. Both starchy foods and sweet foods can raise blood sugar (glucose). But the changes happen at different rates of speed. The rise in blood sugar is more intense if your diet revolves around sweet foods.

Researchers at the University of Toronto got some interesting results when they tested a number of carbohydrates. Pure glucose (dextrose) raised blood sugar fastest and highest. They gave it a "glycemic index" of 100. Sucrose, table sugar, was also high—with an index number of 59. Honey, which releases glucose rapidly, was somewhere in-between. It's glycemic index is 87.

Teaspoon for teaspoon, fructose—a fruit sugar—is roughly twice as sweet as regular sugar. But its glycemic index is only 20. In other words, if you eat fructose instead of sugar or honey, you help avoid the "crash" of low blood sugar (hypoglycemia) that can occur about an hour after you eat. No wonder that, in double-blind testing, fructose helped subjects feel satisfied even when they'd eaten much less food.

The actual experiment went like this: Subjects were given drinks that held an equal number of calories of fructose and sucrose. An hour later, they were allowed to go to a cafeteria and take as much as they wanted to eat. In the study, researchers discovered that those who got the fructose-containing drink ate far less food than those who got sugar-laden drinks instead. Conclusion: If you want the best sweetener in your dessert, have fructose instead of other kinds. (In the dessert recipes in this book, I always recommend fructose as the sweetener of choice.)

ᕯHE SUGAR IN FRUIT

Fruits have a lot of natural sugar in them, so they definitely raise blood sugar. The sweeter the fruit, the less dilution of its sugar among other nutrients, and the higher the glycemic index.

Bananas and raisins are high, at 62 and 64, respectively. Apples and oranges are lower, with a glycemic index of 39 and 40, respectively.

STARCH INDICES

Foods eaten for their complex carbohydrates are not all created equal in glycemic index either. White rice and bread (even whole-wheat bread) are highest at 72, followed by white potatoes at 70. Brown rice is scarcely better at 66. Pasta is notably lower—50 for white spaghetti and 42 for whole-wheat spaghetti. Sweet potatoes and yams are surprisingly low for their sweetness, at 48 and 51.

Last, some vegetables raise blood sugar surprisingly fast and let it crash soon thereafter. Carrots, amazingly, have a glycemic index of 92, nearly as high as pure glucose. So having a bagful of carrots is not a great idea for a snack.

You want food that stays for a while in the stomach and small intestine. As soon as the starches get digested to simple sugars there, they should get absorbed. Otherwise, bacteria in the colon steal the sugars from you, ferment them, and produce carbon dioxide and methane. Digest your food slowly, and the absorptive surface of your small intestine will sop it up like a paper towel, absorbing it all for you. Eat lots of sugar and you get trouble. That's spelled g-a-s.

What's more, slow absorption of sugars from the intestine makes the insulin-secreting cells of your pancreas respond more slowly. To understand this, let's look at the opposite situation—say, when you're eating lots of sugar. As soon as that sugar gets absorbed into the bloodstream, the pancreas gets the word, and says, "Uh-oh, high blood sugar! Bad for the eyes, kidneys, and arteries! Better do something, or we'll get damaged blood vessels in lots of important places."

That's when your pancreas cranks out a monumental amount of insulin. Insulin copes with the sugar overload by making your muscles, fat cells, and liver slurp up the sugar. The muscles and liver make their own storage starch, called glycogen. And guess what the fat cells make? That's right, f-a-t.

Too much starch can also make you fat. But at least starch can't make you fat quickly, and you'll feel hungry less often eating it, so you've got double protection against gaining weight.

$\mathcal{M}$ORE STARCH BENEFITS

There's another benefit to eating starch: It can help you feel full sooner because it holds water.

But watch your step on this one. A single tablespoon of cornstarch can make four full ounces, half a cup, of water into a thick gel. That ratio is okay. Your stomach can cope with mixing a gel and sending it to your intestine.

Something else happens, however, when you eat a dry starch that can absorb more water in your stomach. It stays solid, but it gets bigger and bigger. Think of what happens to dry spaghetti when it goes into boiling water. As in the pasta pot, so in your stomach. Eating too much dry starch (such as bread) without having enough fluid in your system is just like cooking spaghetti without enough boiling water. The spaghetti can't mix, and it sticks together. Result: an uncomfortable lump in your stomach. You will not like this when you go to bed.

I think it's advisable for most of us to eat more starchy foods than we do. But we must be careful of how much we eat, especially late in the evening.

I don't advocate drinking a lot of fluids with dinner, either to wash down the meal or to fill up on water. That will only worsen your digestion by diluting your digestive enzymes. Instead, I recommend that you eat slowly, and with plenty of chewing, so you mix enough saliva with your food. That way, you actually start digesting your food the instant it's in your mouth.

I recommend from experience that you drink only sips of liquid with your meals. Avoid fluids for an hour before and an hour after meals. That will give your stomach some relief in mixing, grinding, and digesting food.

Your stomach is an excellent food processor. Its contractions smash everything down to 1 mm (about 1/25 inch). Your stomach will send that mashed-up food along to the small intestine. That won't take forever if you give it a mixture that it can handle: well-chewed food reasonably well mixed with your digestive secretions.

If you chew plenty, it helps you to eat more slowly, of course. This, too, is important for GERDy people.

Most of us just keep eating until we feel satisfied. But the feeling of satiety is triggered by hormones, and the hormones aren't released right away. First, the food goes to the stomach. That signals the gastrointestinal tract to produce cholecystokinin (CCK). Then this hormone makes the gallbladder contract, bringing useful emulsifiers into your small intestine, and helping you dissolve and digest fats.

CCK has another important function: It sends an "I'm full" satiety signal to the brain via the bloodstream. This is called a "feedback loop" by biochemists. The trouble is, it takes close to half an hour for this feedback from the GI tract to effectively reach the brain.

During that half hour, the gut steadily pumps out CCK, increasing the blood-level concentrations until, finally, we get the brain message that tells us to stop eating. Meantime, we may overeat if we eat fast, as most Americans do. Or we may overeat if we watch TV, read, or talk while we eat and don't pay attention to how we feel. Finally, a common cause of overeating is drinking alcohol before and during a meal. Alcohol essentially dulls our attention, so the satiety signals don't even get through.

Eating slowly makes your food taste tastier. It's very tranquil, very *Zen*. Give the carbohydrates a chance to help you feel full when you are full.

Chapter 8

*F*ATS YOU WANT—
AND SOME
YOU DON'T

*W*hat's the trouble with "no-fat" eating?

Let's go back to the CCK feedback loop for a minute—the one that sends you the signal that you're full. There's another potential problem with it.

I said that CCK was produced when we've had enough to eat. That was oversimplifying. The hormone is produced mainly in response to *fatty* foods. Eat virtually no fat, as recommended in some cardiac diets, and your GI tract will respond by producing little CCK.

With small amounts of the hormone being produced, very little entering the bloodstream, and even less reaching the brain, you may *never* feel satisfied, no matter how much fat-free food you eat. Ever notice that when snacking on pretzels? You eat and eat and it never seems to be enough?

Okay, that's frustrating, but it gets worse. If your CCK output doesn't crank up, your gallbladder won't be stimulated by CCK to empty.

"So what?" you might say. "The gallbladder only secretes bile. That's just needed to help digest fat."

The problem is that you're more likely to get gallstones if your gallbladder isn't emptying as regularly or thoroughly as it should. Eat no fat, and bile never gets squeezed out of the gallbladder, meal after meal, month after month. But the liver keeps making the bile salts that go into bile. The salts keep dripping down to the gallbladder. They get more concentrated, they precipitate, and the precipitation leads to the formation of gallstones.

$\mathcal{L}$OW-FAT, NOT NO-FAT

I don't advocate recipes that are fat-free. The recipes in this book are low-fat, so you'll get 15 to 20 percent of your calories as fat. For a 150-pound person who exercises moderately for half an hour a day, as a recent council on exercise suggests, 30 to 40 grams of daily fat is a reasonable goal. For a 120-pound moderately active woman, 25 to 30 grams of fat a day is the target. Then our livers and gallbladders will be free to produce and secrete as they may.

There's something else you should note about low-fat eating: It helps in losing weight. That's not the subject of this book, but if you want to lose weight, keeping your exercise level up while you decrease your fat intake will certainly do it. (It works, that is, as long as you don't compensate by packing in nonfat foods.)

If you want to lose weight, try keeping your fat intake down to 25 grams a day for a few months. You won't have to alter your eating routine much if you've already found recipes here that you like, and that your stomach likes. Just don't starve your body of fat for six months or a year, okay? Gallstones can be "silent" and dormant and innocent. Or they can hurt terribly, and they can cause life-threatening illness.

With a low-fat diet, you'll get the good results that are sure to come along when you lower your fat intake. If your diet derives 15 to 20 precent of calories from fat, your cholesterol is likely to drop a bit—probably by about 5 percent. That low-fat diet also helps you keep your blood pressure down by keeping your weight down.

$\mathcal{B}$AD FATS

Fat has gotten a bad rap lately. Saturated fats took the first hit. They contribute to high cholesterol and heart disease. We switched from whole milk to skim milk, from butter to margarine, and from Crisco to safflower oil.

Then polyunsaturated fats became enemies too. We switched from safflower, soybean, and corn oil to canola and olive oil. Finally, all fat seemed to be the enemy, and we switched to tasteless no-fat margarine and no-fat processed foods, rubbery cheese, and dry cookies.

True enough, a lot of the fat in our diets is bad for us. Saturated fat does contribute to heart disease.

Butter is highly saturated, and so are cheese, whole milk, and ice cream. The fat in beef is so saturated that it is a solid at room temperature, not an oil. It's so solid that it used to be made into tallow candles.

High intakes of polyunsaturated fats raise cholesterol levels and contribute to heart disease too. You can't just substitute polyunsaturated oils for butter and keep frying everything you eat. Our good old American diet—which means getting about 40 percent of our calories from fat—is quite simply a killer. But this is not the whole story. The fact is, we have a vital need for fats, but they need to be certain kinds.

ℒOW-FAT EATING

Getting 20 percent of your calories from fat does not mean that fat forms one-fifth of the weight of the food. You can't have one tablespoon of olive oil on four tablespoons of cooked pasta and get a 20 percent fat diet. Yes, by weight, that would be 20 percent fat; but by calories, it would be about 70 percent fat!

Here's why. Fat generally comes "straight," undiluted by water (except in milk). It's a little less dense than water, but still, fat, oil, butter, or plain margarine cost a whopping 100 to 120 calories per tablespoon.

Now, the 20 percent fat diet has 20 percent of the *calories* as fat. So a tablespoon of olive oil would have to be served on 400 calories worth of plain pasta. Pasta, typical of starchy foods, is hydrated—plumped up with water—before it is eaten.

Four hundred calories of dry pasta become a whole pound of cooked pasta. You have to eat all of the pasta, a whole pint's worth, with that one tablespoon of olive oil to keep fat intake down to 20 percent of calories.

Look at it another way. How much butter can you put on a slice of bread and get a 20 percent fat-calories snack? Plain white bread has about 70 calories a slice. So you can put about 18 calories worth of butter on it. That's about half a teaspoon.

Have you ever put a half-teaspoon of butter on a whole slice of bread? Try it some time, and you are apt to find it's pretty meager fare. Rather dry.

So, we are going to pick and choose how that 20 percent accumulates in our diet during the day. We're not going to waste our allowance of fat on bakery goods chock-full of oil and fat. There's no point in squandering our fat allowance on hidden fats when we can use our fat intake for two important goals: survival and pleasure.

GOOD FATS

There is a vital need for certain kinds of fat in our bodies. Unfortunately, few of the fat-containing foods that are easily available in supermarkets contain the fatty acids that help keep our membranes whole and our chemical messengers in balance. And unless we have those "good fats," we get deficiency syndromes.

The best-known human deficiency syndromes are the ones that result from a lack of vitamins. For instance, we get scurvy if we eat too little Vitamin C. Scurvy used to kill sailors who ate a diet without fruit month after month. The British Navy found it could prevent scurvy by making sailors eat limes, whence the name "limey." Similarly, rickets results from a lack of Vitamin D, beri-beri results from a lack of thiamin, and so on. These classic deficiency diseases were discovered about a hundred years ago.

The fat-deficiency syndromes are more subtle and are not as well-charted in humans as the vitamin deficiencies. Fortunately, we do know a lot about two essential fat components. We know that lack of *linoleic acid* (LA) in the diet can lead to eczema-like skin eruptions and a dozen other physical problems, including miscarriages. And lack of *alpha-linolenic acid* (ALA) causes still more subtle problems, including neurological and behavioral changes.

Scientists have traced fatty acid requirements in animals. When a young, growing lab rat is deprived of LA and ALA, almost immediately, the animal shows physical signs of fat deficiency. For obvious reasons, such experiments can never be performed on humans, so our exact requirements for the fatty acids are unknown.

Udo Erasmus, an authority on fatty acid requirements, estimates that the minimum daily adult requirement to prevent deficiency syndromes is 3 to 6 grams of LA a day. Erasmus estimates that about one-fifth to half that amount of ALA is required by humans. He recommends as optimal that we eat 9 to 18 grams of LA and 2 to 9 grams of ALA a day.

In drastic cardiac diets, people eat as little as 12 grams of fat a day. Yet, the sources of fat in our diet that have the most essential fatty acids are only about half LA and ALA. So the most essential fatty acids we could get on a 12-gram fat diet would be 6 grams. In other words, if you go on a diet in which fat is drastically reduced, you might get enough LA and ALA to prevent deficiency syndromes, but just barely. You certainly wouldn't be getting an optimal amount of essential fatty acids.

How can we satisfy our need for essential fatty acids and still be good to our hearts? Certain fats are good for us when consumed in moderation. In addition to LA and ALA, the essential *polyunsaturated* fatty acids, there's another group that has been called "good *monounsaturated* fatty acids" or just good monounsaturates.

Sources of good monounsaturated fatty acids are easy to find nowadays: They're olive and canola oil. Make these the backbone of your fat intake, and you get a high proportion of good monounsaturated fatty acid, called *oleic* acid. This helps you avoid heart attacks and strokes by keeping your cholesterol down.

Canola, but not olive, oil can provide another benefit. About 30 percent of fresh canola oil is comprised of the essential fatty acid LA, while another 7 percent is made up of that other essential fatty acid, ALA.

Because of their complex chemical structure, the molecules in these fatty acids slip around one another easily. They melt at lower temperatures and aggregate differently than saturated fatty acids do. So they're oils at room temperature—not solid, like butter or tallow—and they help our membranes to be more elastic.

We need fatty acids like LA and ALA to form prostaglandins and other master-messengers that control how cells function. That's part of why they're so essential.

It takes some effort when eating a low-fat diet to get enough of the essential fatty acids and to get the right proportion of them, so that they work together effectively. They're too diluted in most fats that we're familiar with. Worse, the processing of oils, refining them so they are clear and nearly colorless, kills their essential fatty acids.

It's the price of all that polyunsaturation. It makes oils subject to damage by heat and air, by the oxygen in the air.

If you want to see this oxygenation process in action, consider what happens to paint that's made with linseed oil. Just one day out in the air, and the polyunsaturated oil in flax-seed (linseed) oil-based housepaint gets polymerized by the air to a tough gel that resists sun and water for years.

In food, any exposure to air does the same thing—ruins the polyunsaturates. This unfortunately is what happens to the LA and ALA in ordinary commercial processing of oils. They get overheated, exposed to air, and then filtered. They come out clear and sanitary, but that clear, sanitary condition is not the best for providing essential fatty acids.

Good commercial sources of essential fatty acids do exist, however. Raw, unroasted, untoasted fresh nut meats are fine sources. So are fresh, cool-pressed oils. Hain makes a whole line of them, called *expeller-pressed* oils. Buy fresh expeller-pressed canola oil, keep it covered tightly, and keep it in the refrigerator.

For variety, try other expeller-pressed oils. The oil from walnuts and wheat germ has as much as 50 percent LA and 5 percent ALA. Soybean oil is similar. (But soybean oil has less of the good monounsaturates, the oleic acid, so my preference is canola.) Olive oil is also beneficial when it comes to supplying essential fatty acids; but while it donates LA, it has no ALA.

Consider the Fat Pleasures

Now for the pleasures of fat. Fat can be a lot more fun than just to lubricate a donut into sliding down the throat. Yes, fat provides a pleasing, soft texture to foods. Also, some of it adds good flavor. Butter, for instance, provides a combination of sweetness, cheese-like taste, and tartness. Beef and chicken fat seem to bring out the essence of their respective meats' taste.

But these three bad actors in heart disease are not essential to get any or all of these tastes. The breadspread recipe in this book provides each of the pleasures of butter. The hyped beef or chicken flavor provided by their fats can also be evoked by adding bouillon crystals in higher than usual concentration and "salting" recipes with flavor enhancers. One is NuSalt, a judicious mix of salt substitute (potassium chloride) and potassium glutamate, a flavor enhancer. Another fine flavor enhancer is Bragg Liquid Aminos, a soy hydrolyzate that has glutamate in it in a solution that tastes salty yet has moderate amounts of salt in it.

One goal of this book is to help you not miss saturated fats. The tricks just mentioned will go a long way toward this goal. Try them and see for yourself.

Chapter 9

$\mathcal{T}$HE PROTEIN FACTOR

$\mathcal{W}$e have been lectured to almost all our lives to eat more protein. Meat, milk, eggs, and cheese—those are the building blocks of good growth and good health. "You never outgrow your need for milk." "You have to eat all your meat before you can have any dessert!"

Well, that was wrong. There's an outside chance that your kidneys may have to work too hard to get rid of all the nitrogen in a high-protein diet. There's a good chance that protein makes you fat. And it's as sure as can be that eating all that protein is unnecessary.

Our protein requirements are much lower than previously proclaimed by the USDA, the department that issues dietary guidelines.

Instead of 100 grams a day or 70 grams a day, all that adults require is 30 grams a day, as in one dish of whole-grain cereal and a serving of beans or peas. This gives us all the protein constituents, the *essential amino acids*, needed to prevent imbalances for a whole day. That's right; no milk, cheese, meat, or eggs are needed.

Recently, it's been found that even broccoli is a better source of protein (calorie for calorie) than meat! How can this be?

Let's go back to biochemistry. Protein molecules are like very long charm bracelets, with a hundred or even a thousand "charms" per molecule. There are only about twenty kinds of charms (amino acids), no matter how big the protein. Each charm hangs from a link of chain and is forged to it more tightly than the links of chain are hooked together.

When you eat protein, your digestive enzymes (starting with saliva) work on that protein. They hydrolyze the connections between the links of chain. This frees the amino acids. Then the amino acids get absorbed by the intestinal lining.

So, it doesn't matter how much the protein source resembles your body. That isn't what makes it good protein. What makes it good protein is only the composition of the amino acids that are released from it by digestion.

Among the amino acids that are released, the most important are the essential amino acids. These are the eight that we can't make by converting other amino acids in the liver.

Some proteins are not balanced enough. Gelatin is abundant in only three of the twenty amino acids! Corn protein lacks the essential amino acid lysine. Most cereals are low in protein (about 10%), and their balance of the essential amino acids isn't good enough. But supplementing them with legumes (beans, peas, or peanuts) gives a good balance of amino acids.

So, let's put high-protein animal foods in their place. They are interesting, toothsome, chewy flavors, but not staples. Eat none of them, though, and you may feel deprived if you are accustomed to having meat in your daily diet.

But don't think you have to make protein a big part of your dinner in order to leave the table feeling full and satisfied. Beef doesn't have to be the heart of the meal; you don't have to serve meat as the item to fill up on. It is not written anywhere that meat must be served as a big slab in the middle of the plate. A single ounce of good lean meat can make a Chinese meal satisfying.

ᐃHAT'S NEEDED—WHAT'S NOT

Another controversy is heating up about protein requirements. That controversy relates to the glycemic index that I discussed earlier.

Maybe you thought only carbohydrate-containing foods have a glycemic index—that they were the only foods that could raise blood glucose.

Not so! Most of the amino acids released from high-protein foods can be converted into glucose by the liver when protein intake is in excess of the minimum required to keep amino acid levels adequate in the body. But this should mean that high-protein foods have a low glycemic index, right? Because they must be digested and processed in the liver before they can form any glucose, eating more protein should lower the glycemic index of our meals.

As I've mentioned, the lower the glycemic index of a food, the less it raises your blood sugar and your insulin levels. This is true not only of fruits, vegetables, and carbohydrate foods. It's also true of the high-protein foods. Plain yogurt, for instance, typical of dairy products, has a glycemic index of only 36, lower than any of the complex carbohydrate foods like rice, potatoes, or bread.

Soybeans, the protein champs of the legumes, have a glycemic index of only 15. Fish and meats are low, too. Even a sweetened meat product like sausage has a glycemic index of only 28.

More important, it's the *overall* glycemic index of the meal that counts more than the glycemic index of any one component. A snack of a cup of plain yogurt (glycemic index 36), even with a teaspoon of honey (glycemic index 87), still has a low overall glycemic index. So adding more protein to meals may help you avoid hunger a couple of hours after eating, even if it is not absolutely required to replace bodily amino acids burned away by metabolism.

Adding high-protein foods does another good deed. It stimulates release of glucagon from the pancreas into your bloodstream. Glucagon acts in opposition to insulin, raising blood sugar from stored glycogen and mobilizing fat from fat cells. So you not only don't feel hungry two hours after a meal, you feel good because you have adequate energy for thinking and doing.

So, what protein level should we shoot for? It's not clear yet. The Recommended Dietary Allowance (RDA) of 30 grams a day is less than 10 percent of calories. Even cereal has more protein than this.

For hard-training athletes, a 30 percent (of calories) protein diet is now recommended. Until the experts can tell us non-varsity athletes how much protein to eat, the data on heart disease convinces me to continue eating as little high-protein food as I can. I'm going to eat just enough so that I feel satisfied.

My high-protein food sources will continue to be those with the least possible fat, especially saturated fat. That means limiting meats to the very heart-healthiest. If you're going to eat chicken, I recommend white meat without skin. Avoid red meats, except for the occasional ounce of lean pork to flavor a mixed dish.

There's really no reason to eat processed meats, but if you do, try low-fat, smoked turkey products in amounts only sufficient to flavor mixed dishes.

In my own diet, I eat lean fish a couple of times a week. Among dairy products, I look for nonfat versions like nonfat cottage cheese and yogurt. I eat egg whites or egg substitutes instead of eggs. And instead of meat, I prefer high-protein vegetable foods such as low-fat tofu, beans, veggie burgers, and not-dogs.

If I feel hungry between meals, it will be a snack with a low overall glycemic index for me: an apple or half a cup of nonfat yogurt with a teaspoon or two of fructose, some sliced fruit, and maybe some cinnamon or wheat germ or vanilla.

Chapter 10

GETTING YOUR VITAMINS AND MINERALS

True or false: A pill can give you all the vitamins known to science.

Well, it's true, but it's also misleading.

Science knows all the organic cofactors that we cannot manufacture for ourselves that are needed for basic metabolism. In fact, that's a good description of the vitamins that we know a lot about: They're organic molecules that help our enzymes catalyze chemical reactions in our bodies.

But science is just scratching the surface of knowledge of all the organic cofactors needed for some subtle, hidden biochemical processes that ward off cancer and other diseases of later adulthood. Antioxidants, flavonoids, carotenoids, terpenes, sesquiterpenes, lycopenes, polyphenols. . . the list of new nutritional heroes seems to grow longer every month.

However, the number of *sources* of all these compounds doesn't get long. All of those compounds, plus many more, are found in common plants that we eat.

Some of the recent scientific literature suggests that we need to eat several sorts of vegetables and fruits to get these cofactors into our bodies and keep enough of them to benefit the most from them. It's the same old list that Mama taught us: leafy greens, yellow or orange vegetables, and whole grains and vegetables with plenty of roughage.

As my professors at the University of Wisconsin taught me, if you want to find a new cofactor for better growth or protection from diseases, just grind up some spinach and start testing and purifying. Of course, there are many more eligible greens than just spinach. The best salads include many of them—kale, beet greens, chicory, endive, and even dandelion greens.

The yellow vegetables like cauliflower, carrots, and tomatoes have their own contributions to make to our nutritional needs. Carrots are, not surprisingly, the best common source of carotenes.

Carrots also suggest a subversive, politically incorrect idea: Cooking may be good for your health. Cooking carrots increases the availability of the carotenes for absorption. (This is not to say, however, that cooking *always* increases the nutritional value of our food to us. I generally recommend cooking things minimally, not only because the most flavor is evoked this way or because it takes the least time, but also because some vitamins are destroyed by heating.)

You may have read that microwave cooking destroys vitamins, for instance. If you cook vegetables the way the microwave instruction books say, on "High" for the whole process, you will scorch away some of the vitamins. Also, cooking this way saves little time compared to heating veggies to boiling and then continuing to heat them at the boiling point (simmering them), either in a two-stage microwave or on the range.

There are at least four ways you can effectively cook vegetables without depleting their nutrients. In addition to using the microwave, you can gently simmer, stir-fry, sauté, and steam them.

$\mathcal{B}$ARING FRUIT

Fruits are increasingly being found to contribute more than just sugar and other carbohydrates to our diets. Strawberries, for instance, are packed with the soluble fiber that is so good for lowering cholesterol. Half a cup has more fiber than a bowlful of oatmeal, and strawberries have lycopenes in high quantity. These rather newly appreciated antioxidants may be important to ward off the degenerative diseases of old age. Unfortunately, the USDA allows so much pesticide use on strawberries that you can taste it. Better buy organic.

Apples are an outstanding source of one of the flavonoids. This is another class of antioxidants that protect from atherosclerosis and other degenerative diseases. Yellow and orange fruits get their color from carotenes, sources of Vitamin A and also great antioxidants.

Some fruits even have exotic organic cofactors in them that are found nowhere else. Bromelain in pineapple is one of these cofactors.

Or they may have helpful digestants, like the protein-digesting enzyme papain in papaya.

Fruits are certainly good sources of many needed minerals. Bananas and oranges, for instance, are especially rich in potassium.

In general, fruits are now considered as important as vegetables to ensure good nutrition. They can't replace leafy greens, but they are important in their own right. In total, you should try to get close to a dozen servings of fruit and vegetables every day.

A few tropical fruits contain high proportions of saturated fats. There are no recipes in this book employing coconut or avocado. This is not an unconditional censure, however. Small quantities of these fruits will not hurt you any more than saturated fat from butter does.

REAL MINERAL REQUIREMENTS AND TOXIC MINERALS

MINERALS BY THE GRAM

The big four nutritional minerals are calcium, sodium, potassium, and magnesium. That is, we get a lot of them compared to the other minerals. There's only one bad actor in this cast of characters: sodium. Let's check it out first.

Sodium in the diet does little good for us, except to magnify the tastes of foods. Our cells need sodium, but mostly outside the cell membrane. In fact, cells have special pumps to keep most of the sodium out.

We need sodium in the blood, to maintain its tonicity, and we need it in all the fluids that bathe our cells. Bathe cells in fluids with too little sodium and they lose their minerals and swell up, just the way skin gets milky-looking and puckers when exposed to plain water for too long. But we need little or no sodium in our *diets*, because our kidneys are great at keeping the sodium that we already have in our bodies. Even our sweat adapts over time. If we consume less sodium, our perspiration is less salty.

Sodium is very hard to avoid in the diet. Most soups are very high in sodium, several grams per serving, and you can usually taste the saltiness. But did you know that most breads are also high in sodium?

Or would you expect that milk, cheese, and even cottage cheese are high in sodium? So are commercial hamburgers, fried or roasted chicken, and Chinese and Italian foods.

In fact, everything produced commercially, except a few select items such as salads and baked potatoes, has sodium. (Even salads have sky-high sodium content if you eat them with salad dressing.) It's usual for Americans to consume 10 grams of sodium a day.

Some Japanese people consume even more. Coastal villagers consume up to 40 grams of sodium a day. Their rates of stroke are astronomical.

American diets, with their high levels of sodium, also cause cardiovascular disease. They are linked to high blood pressure, which is as bad for your arteries as smoking is. It damages the inside of the artery wall directly. Inflammation starts there, and fatty bubbles can break off, causing sudden damage where they plug smaller arteries such as coronaries. The artery tries to protect itself by applying patches to the damaged spots. But the patches grow, become fibrous, and act like tumors, growing locally as they take on globs of cholesterol. This is atherosclerosis, the other killer in heart attacks and strokes.

High blood pressure is virtually nonexistent in cultures where sodium intake is very low. Trouble is, if you eat consistently with the dominant culture, you'd have to be a native in the Amazon rainforest or a farmhand in Asia to bring your sodium intake down to levels that don't cause hypertension.

You can defy the cultural norms here in America and cut your blood pressure by avoiding sodium, but you would probably have to eat as little as 500 milligrams of it per day to do so. This is equivalent to only about 1.3 grams of salt.

To achieve this you'd have to find salt-free bread or bake your own; eat no fast-foods or restaurant fare; take in no prepared food from the frozen foods section of the supermarket; and eat no dairy products.

The usual low-sodium diet prescribed for people with hypertension or kidney disease is comprised of 2 to 4 grams of salt a day. Such diets have recently been shown not to lower blood pressure appreciably in patients with hypertension.

Yet we are in the midst of an epidemic of hypertension. Fifteen to 25 percent of the adult male population has it, depending on what cultural or racial group is counted.

One study showed that a sodium-restricted diet was associated with a higher risk of heart attacks. The conclusion was that too much sodium restriction resulted in oversecretion of a hormone called renin, which raises the blood pressure and helps the body retain sodium when needed. Yet another recent study showed that sodium restriction increased the incidence of kidney stones.

What can you do, practically speaking?

First, you can keep your sodium intake down to reasonable levels, more than 4 and less than 10 grams a day, so you don't risk stroke or hypertension. To maintain the lower level of sodium intake, avoid fast-food places and pre-prepared foods.

It's a great help if you can cook for yourself. Cooking at home, without using a lot of prepared foods, you can easily keep your sodium intake down to the vicinity of 4 grams to avoid development of hypertension.

Also, you can replace much of the sodium in the usual American high-sodium diet with a salt substitute. Add potassium to your diet and you can have the flavor enhancement without the hypertension.

Most of the recipes in this book suggest cooking with fresh ingredients, and the recipes are created so that you can eat within half an hour of the time you start preparing to cook. In fact, it's so quick and easy to cook meals at home that the term "fast food" is generally misleading. By the time you drive to a restaurant, wait in line at the window or counter, and drive back home, you can easily prepare a simple, low-sodium, low-fat meal that will cost less, taste better, and guard your cardiovascular system from all kinds of trouble.

Potassium is a vital ingredient in our diets, and we need a lot of it, 3500 milligrams a day according to the RDA. Normal kidneys do not retain potassium well, the way they do sodium. A great deal of potassium can be lost in sweat. This used to put athletes and manual laborers at risk of heat prostration, until the advent of Gatorade and other products that replenish potassium losses.

Potassium is actively pumped into all of our cells, balancing the tonicity outside the cells that is produced by sodium. The proper concentration must be maintained in the blood within pretty narrow limits, or the heart muscle cannot maintain a life-preserving rhythm.

Fortunately, potassium is present in many foods. Some vegetables are quite high in it, especially potatoes. Milk products are fairly high in potassium too. So is orange juice. Many people recognize that bananas are a great source of potassium, but fewer know that tea is also an excellent source.

As a rule, the more we get away from natural foods and exist on pre-prepared foods, the lower our intake of potassium. Meat, bread, pasta, and rice are so-so in potassium content. Fats, oils, and sugar don't have any of it.

Potassium is a natural blood pressure medicine. The amount required to lower blood pressure by 5 to 10 points is about the same as if you cook with a salt substitute and sprinkle it on food. So that is exactly what this book's recipes ask you to do.

Salt substitutes are usually potassium chloride, KCl. If you try a plain one, you may find it causes an irritating, almost burning feeling on your tongue, and seems bitter. But you might be using too much. Before you give up on it, try using less on each serving. Its effect seems more concentrated than that of table salt.

Also, try the KCl on various foods. It's better tasting on some foods than others.

Generally, I look for Nu Salt brand, or any brand with some potassium glutamate in it. This seems to make it all the more concentrated in its saltiness and, for me at least, eliminates the bitterness.

Not all salt substitutes are KCl. Some are herb mixes, such as Mrs. Dash. Be careful with these, however, as they may irritate the stomach. Dried garlic, onion, and red pepper are frequent ingredients.

Calcium is in short supply in our diets. We're warned about osteoporosis if we don't drink enough milk. The RDA for calcium is 1000 milligrams, and that requires three eight-ounce glasses of milk a day.

Recent research in postmenopausal women has shown that a calcium supplement supplying 1700 milligrams a day along with twice the RDA for Vitamin D cut bone mineral loss. Likewise, a French study of elderly women found that similar supplements cut the incidence of hip fractures.

Another study, of younger men, showed that increasing the calcium intake to about 1500 milligrams daily decreased LDL (bad cholesterol) in the blood by 11 percent, by increasing fecal excretion rather than systemic effects.

A National Institutes of Health Consensus Conference in 1994 recommended an adult daily calcium intake of 1000 to 1500 milligrams.

How are we going to consume all that calcium? A cup of milk or yogurt or two ounces of cheese, cottage cheese, or fat-free cream cheese has about 300 milligrams of calcium, a third of the minimum RDA. We're encouraged to eat canned tuna and salmon, bones and all (100 milligrams of calcium in ¼ cup).

Tofu provides calcium, and so do some vegetables. You'll get 100 milligrams of calcium from half a cup of tofu, cooked white beans, or greens.

Some juices and milk substitutes are spiked with calcium. You'll get 300 milligrams in each cup of calcium-fortified orange juice or cup of milk substitute.

But keep in mind that calcium *balance* is the key issue, not calcium *intake*. For starters, calcium intake does not equal calcium absorption.

Without good supplies of the active metabolites of Vitamin D produced by your body, you will not absorb calcium from the diet. You need at least 400 international units of Vitamin D for this. Then, at least in the normal circumstance, several hormonal systems carefully balance calcium intake, calcium use in bones, and calcium output in urine.

Vitamin D metabolites and the hormones calcitonin and thyrocalcitonin collectively control buildup and breakdown of calcium in bone, and retention or loss of calcium from the kidney.

Postmenopausal women have a hormonal system that may cause a negative calcium balance in the body, causing them to lose more calcium than they absorb every day. Men and premenopausal women are likely to have less daily calcium loss. So the calcium requirements for postmenopausal women is generally higher than for males and younger women.

However, there is one other important way to keep calcium in your bones: with *exercise.*

Calcium balance changes radically when people do not exercise. Bedridden patients fall rapidly into negative calcium balance. Even robust astronauts lose calcium when they are in the weightless conditions of space. So beware, couch potatoes: A sedentary lifestyle is hazardous to your bones!

Engaging in weight training for a year, on the other hand, increases bone density, even in postmenopausal women. The key is apparently to put compressive strains on bones, because weight lifting is the best known way to increase bone density.

Magnesium may be vital for the heart. Clinical data implicate low levels of magnesium in heart disease. Patients with heart attacks or coronary artery disease have low levels of free (unbound to protein) magnesium in their blood.

Also, population data suggest that low magnesium is linked to heart disease. The incidence of death from cardiovascular diseases in the eastern U.S. is significantly higher than in the west, where there tends to be more magnesium in the water.

Studies show that humans and other animals have increased atherosclerosis if they have low levels of magnesium in their blood and diets. Low magnesium levels also cause spasm of arteries, which can cause angina pectoris, the chest pain from a choked blood supply to the heart. Low magnesium intake causes hypertension, which contributes to atherosclerosis.

There is also considerable evidence that magnesium is necessary to avoid diabetes and migraine.

Now comes the bad news: Our diets are poor in magnesium. Daily intake of magnesium is about 170 to 260 milligrams a day, compared to the RDA of 350 milligrams a day. Worse yet, experts believe that the RDA is too low and should be 450 to 500 milligrams a day, which was the typical daily intake around the year 1900.

The good news is that our water may supply all we need, but that's wildly variable depending on the source of the water. Meltwater from snow on mountains is very low in magnesium, so the folks who drink its runoff in places such as Portland, Oregon get precious little magnesium in their water.

Contrast that with the water supply in many areas of Michigan, where water percolates through limestone, picking up minerals as it goes. There, the water is so full of calcium and magnesium that it clogs pipes and stains sinks. So people soften their water, replacing the magnesium and calcium with sodium. The irony is, people in Michigan may get as little magnesium in their water as the people in Portland do.

Drink hard water or get heart disease? Clearly, more options are needed.

A vegetarian diet is associated with a low incidence of heart disease and hypertension and with above-average levels of magnesium intake. Legumes, beans, nuts, soybeans, green leafy veggies, and whole grains are rich in magnesium. Of course, fats, oils, and sugar—processed foods in general—are low in magnesium.

I'll take my chances on using some meats to add interest to my diet, but I wouldn't do without the ingredients of a vegetable diet that add magnesium. And, just to be sure, I take 300 milligrams of magnesium in an absorbable supplement. (An amino acid chelate such as magnesium aspartate is better absorbed than magnesium sulfate or magnesium oxide.)

There's one characteristic of magnesium supplements that needs mentioning: They can cause diarrhea. Unless your bowels run slowly, don't try replacing your magnesium shortfall with milk of magnesia (magnesium hydroxide).

MINERALS BY THE MILLIGRAM

Many minerals are needed in milligram or even microgram quantities daily. It's beyond the scope of this book to discuss all of them and their requirements. A few notes are included here to alert you to the importance of getting enough of two of them through (mostly vegetable) sources or supplements.

A leading expert on **zinc** advised me that it may be the most limiting micromineral in the diet. Just how low a level of zinc creates a deficiency is hard to define, because the signs and symptoms may be subtle in people who eat ordinary diets.

Zinc is marginal in the U.S. diet; we typically get 12 to 15 of the 15 milligrams RDA. Worse for us, the absorption of zinc is prevented by certain chemicals called *chelators*.

There are two main culprits. One is in prepared foods and is called EDTA, which is added as a preservative. The other is phytin, a natural chelator in some vegetables. As with most other nutrients, eating a wide variety of vegetables is the best way to assure adequate zinc intake.

To avoid EDTA on your veggies, read the labels before you buy salad dressings and frozen vegetables, two of the prime sources of this preservative.

Another illustrative example of the importance of eating a variety of ordinary foods is one athlete's experience with **manganese**. Basketball star Bill Walton went on a macrobiotic diet and kept getting leg fractures until he was diagnosed as low in manganese and was treated for it.

Manganese is recognized as a cofactor required for bone formation. Interesting, isn't it? Walton's calcium supply wasn't low, and he obviously got plenty of weight-bearing exercise, which stimulates bone growth, in pro basketball. But he was still unable to maintain the bone he needed to support a very large body structure—all because he didn't eat enough of a subtle cofactor. Once he had enough manganese, the bone knit normally.

Puzzling Minerals

Mineral nutrition may seem old hat, but we have a lot to learn. For instance, **chromium** and **selenium**, toxic except in microgram quantities daily, are apparently important antioxidants.

There has been much discussion of the importance of antioxidants. But which ones are *most* important? Some, such as Vitamin E and beta carotene, are better established than others as important for cardiovascular health.

Until the whole picture emerges, I'll take supplements to make sure I get enough of each antioxidant—and no more—because many a metallic mineral element can be toxic.

Absorption of minerals by the body can be extremely low, contributing to inadequacies. Chromium is not only an antioxidant; it is also important to help keep blood glucose down—it helps insulin.

Our diets seem adequate in raw amounts of chromium, usually containing over 30 micrograms compared to the 1 microgram that we need. But chromium absorption by the body is only about 1 percent or less, so supplements may be important, especially in people with a tendency to diabetes.

Chromium supplements come in 100 micrograms, to cope with the low expected rate of absorption of 1 percent or less.

Quantity seems more important for required minerals than for vitamins. Clearly, **copper, zinc**, and many other micromineral nutrients can be toxic in quantities greater than the RDA. **Iron**, formerly paid slavish homage as vital to everybody, is falling into disfavor, except to keep blood counts up to needed levels in women who are menstruating and in children. Without iron supplements, people in these groups may become anemic.

It's now theorized that iron supplements may actually be harmful to others, because iron is a pro-oxidant, promoting free radical damage in the body.

Toxic Minerals

Perhaps as important as getting the beneficial minerals is avoiding the outright toxic minerals. **Aluminum** has been implicated in Alzheimer's disease, and doctors tell patients with kidney failure, who can't get rid of aluminum, to avoid aluminum-containing antacids and even aluminum cookware.

Every parent is scared of **lead** in paint. Some ceramic glazes are high in lead, so use handmade ceramics for cooking or making tea only if you are sure they are safe. Fishermen should know to consume their catch in limited quantities because of the **mercury** content. Fish that eat other fish are much higher in mercury.

Still other minerals simply puzzle us. A few milligrams of **boron** is touted as good for us in some health food stores. Even **germanium** is promoted. As a nutritional biochemist, I know of no bodily function for either of these elements. Just because they may be important to computer chips doesn't mean they'll help my body process anything better.

Chapter 11

$\mathcal{P}$LANNING
YOUR MENUS

$\mathcal{S}$imple menus are provided here for five small meals a day, with options for vegetarians. Multiple small feedings a day is the goal. For most of us, it is easier to take time for a meal first thing in the morning, at noontime, and early in the evening than at other times.

The other small feedings are aimed for a mid-morning and a mid-afternoon break. This is a small departure from the usual medical advice on diet for GERD and peptic ulcer, which is to eat six small meals a day.

If you eat dinner early enough, you may want or even need another snack later in the evening. Or you might have one of the recommended desserts an hour or two after dinner. Either way, remember not to eat for two hours before bedtime.

After you feel well again and are on a maintenance program of lifestyle modification (and perhaps medication), you may find it easier to revert to three meals a day. The only modifications that will be needed to these menus are to increase the portions at meals and skip the snacks. Still, be guided by your symptoms.

If eating larger meals bothers you, go back to smaller ones and start snacking again.

𝒪𝓂ENUS

Omnivore	**Vegetarian Substitutions**

First Day

Breakfast

Hot oatmeal, brown sugar and raisins, with nonfat milk	Soy, rice, or oatmeal with nonfat milk
Smoked low-fat cheese and whole wheat toast	Baked soy
Hot apple juice with cinnamon stick	

Mid-Morning Snack

Sliced banana, whole wheat pretzels, plain yogurt on cinnamon raisin bagel half

1 tbsp. all-fruit jam

Lunch

Chicken rice soup	Split pea vegetable soup
Whole wheat bread with Promise Ultra margarine	
Green salad with celery seed dressing	
Mineral water with twist of lime	

Mid-Afternoon Snack

Broccoli, cauliflower, and carrot crudités with nonfat sour cream dip whipped with dashes of lemon, salt, and pepper to taste	Dip of Silken tofu

Dinner

Broiled salmon with herbs	Easy mushroom risotto
Microwave-steamed red potatoes	Panned red chard
Panned snow peas	
Oatmeal raisin cookies	

Second Day

Breakfast

Grilled ham slice	Tempeh tots (slice 4 ounces tempeh $1/4$ inch thick, cut into 1-inch squares; fry in 1 tablespoon olive oil until lightly browned)

Omnivore	**Vegetarian Substitutions**

SECOND DAY—*Breakfast* (cont'd)

Hot chunky applesauce
Vanilla yogurt   Tofurella®

Mid-Morning Snack

1–2 ounces canned tuna   Tofu Swiss "cheese"
Health Valley whole wheat crackers

Lunch

Green salad with vinegar and oil

Mid-Afternoon Snack

Plain hummus and pita wedges

Dinner

Fettuccine al burro   Microwaved broccoliflower
Proscuitto or Black Forest ham garnish   with brown and wild
Panned Swiss chard   rice mix
White grape juice
Peach cobbler

THIRD DAY

Breakfast

Total® cereal, nonfat milk, fresh blueberries,
    brown sugar
Oatmeal toast with breadspread

Mid-Morning Snack

Broccoli florets with fat-free sour cream
Whole wheat breadsticks

Lunch

Potato-cheese soup   Greens and beans soup
Whole wheat toast

Mid-Afternoon Snack

Salad of soy nuts, romaine lettuce,
    and raisins with apple cider vinegar

Omnivore	**Vegetarian Substitutions**

THIRD DAY *(cont'd)*

Dinner

Fettuccine a la carbonara with panned kale	Tabouli
Green salad with balsamic vinaigrette	
Whole wheat pita bread	
Vanilla Tofutti®	
Basil-infused olive oil for dipping	
Concord grape juice	

FOURTH DAY

Breakfast

Banana quickbread with breadspread	
Fresh strawberries	
Chilled low-fat milk	Vanilla rice milk

Mid-Morning Snack

Red and green grapes
Oat bran pretzels
Tablespoon of peanut butter

Lunch

Smoked turkey breast sandwich on rye	Smoky baked tofu, sliced with leaf lettuce and sprinkled with olive oil, vinegar, and oregano
Canned peaches in juice	
Mineral water	

Mid-Afternoon Snack

Black bean dip
Whole wheat breadsticks
Oregon Berry juice cocktail

Dinner

Grilled chicken over brown and wild rice	Grilled tempeh
Microwaved butternut squash	
Fruit salad	

Omnivore	**Vegetarian Substitutions**

FIFTH DAY

Breakfast

Cheese-flavored biscuits	Plain biscuits
Grilled lean ground pork spiced as breakfast sausage	Vegetarian "breakfast sausage"

Mid-Morning Snack

Nonfat Swiss cheese	Tofurella®
Whole wheat crackers	

Lunch

Grilled chicken salad	Three-bean salad
Honey-mustard yogurt dressing	
Chilled boiled red potatoes	

Mid-Afternoon Snack

Salad of leaf lettuce, frozen peas,
   and carrot slices with balsamic vinegar
Mineral water

Dinner

Chicken stroganoff	Vegetarian stroganoff
Panned beet tops and low-fat bacon dressing	
Baked Granny Smith apple	

SIXTH DAY

Breakfast

Low-fat hash browns	
Ground turkey breakfast sausage	Morningstar Farm "sausage"
Pear halves grilled with buttery-flavored spray	

Mid-Morning Snack

Pea pods and spinach leaves with low-fat bacon dressing	Vinegar and oil dressing

Lunch

Stir-fried cauliflower
Red grape juice

Omnivore	Vegetarian Substitutions

SIXTH DAY *(cont'd)*

Mid-Afternoon Snack

Plain yogurt with 1 tablespoon
  all-fruit jam

Dinner

Turkey-artichoke white pizza	Mushroom-broccoli pizza
White grape juice	
Dutch apple pie	

SEVENTH DAY

Breakfast

| Whole-grain cereal muffin with all-fruit strawberry jam | |
| Grilled Canadian bacon slice | Melt Tofurella® on the muffin |

Mid-Morning Snack

Toasted cinnamon-raisin bagel half with
  nonfat cream cheese breadspread
Red and green grapes

Lunch

Tuna-Nayonaise® salad sandwich on
  whole wheat bread
Apple
Chilled carrot juice

Mid-Afternoon Snack

Plain yogurt with 2 teaspoons brown
  sugar and dash allspice

Dinner

Broiled mahimahi with coriander
  butter sauce
Steamed baby carrots and snow peas
Brown rice
White grape juice
Cherry cobbler with vanilla yogurt topping

Part 3

$\mathcal{E}$ATING RIGHT FOR A HEALTHY STOMACH

Chapter 12

GROCERY SHOPPING AND STORAGE

Don't pick a recipe and then shop: You'll eat the wrong stuff in the meantime. On the other hand, when you get home tired from the office, grocery shopping is the last thing in the world you'll want to do. Don't settle for eating a dinner that's bad for you. Instead, so you'll be able to cook something you'll want, stock up on the foods listed here each week and keep them in your freezer, fridge, or pantry.

MEAT

Refrigerate meats for 3 days or less, mindful of outdates on the package, or freeze for 6 months or less (6 weeks or less for smoked meats).

➡ boneless pork tenderloin

➡ boneless skinless chicken breasts (Amish, if you can find them—raised without hormones and antibiotics)

➡ low-fat turkey Canadian bacon

➡ low-fat turkey ham

➡ turkey breast, sliced or whole (Amish, if available)

FISH

Keep frozen fish for not more than 6 weeks. Keep fresh fish wrapped and on ice at the freezing point—below refrigerator temperature!—for no more than 24 hours (see salmon recipe).

FIRM FISH

➠ **Salmon, swordfish, tuna, or mahimahi.**

These are firm enough to be easy to handle. They hold up to cooking well; they don't get mushy when overcooked a little. Pacific salmon tastes drier and tougher. Atlantic salmon is much softer. It cooks faster, and can get mushy from overcooking. Its higher content of liquids makes it better served plain than Pacific salmon is.

➠ **Canned water-pack salmon and tuna.**

These vary in taste and other qualities by species. Generally, you get what you pay for. Among salmon, the firmest, pinkest, most flavorful kind is king salmon, also called silver. The lightest, both in color and in taste, is chum, which may also be called silverbright just to confuse you. Tunas vary also.

Don't get me started on tuna terminology; it's too confusing. Albacore tuna, for instance, is falsely named. When you get "albacore tuna," you get a real tuna but a false albacore. A real albacore is not a tuna, but it is a close relative. It is sometimes marketed not as albacore but as "whitemeat tuna."

Pinker stuff may be called "light tuna." It may not be in steaks but instead in chunks. The label should say so. Fresh tuna probably won't have the species on the package label. Check color and firmness; that's what counts.

SOFT FISH

➠ **Catfish, cod, bluefish, grouper, lake perch, orange roughy, rainbow trout, red snapper, sea perch (plaice), tilapia, etc.**

Tending to be lower on the food chain, soft fish are usually lower in heavy metals and other contaminants. Soft fish are amazingly quick-cooking. In the sizes commonly available in the markets, they'll cook in 5 or 6 minutes in a pan. They overcook easily. An overcooked fillet (*fill'-let*, not *fil-eh'*) of soft fish is mushy and repulsive.

Most soft fish are wonderfully adaptive. They take to other flavors easily because they have little flavor of their own. This makes them easily seasoned without resorting to the Cajun overkill method. A few of the soft fishes, especially bluefish, trout, and a few others, have distinctive flavors to be honored. If you don't want a strong taste, don't buy them. The amount of taste varies greatly with the freshness of the fish. Ask the person behind the counter if you have doubts about which to buy or how to cook and season it.

$\mathcal{D}$AIRY PRODUCTS

Switching to nonfat dairy products is easiest done by a process of gradual accommodation. You can go from whole milk (about 3.5 percent butterfat) to 2 percent to 1 percent to skim. Even with cottage cheese, you can go from whole (about 4 percent butterfat) to 2 percent to nonfat. But with cream cheese, it's all or nothing, unless you want to mix products together. And with cheese, you may find that low-fat is as far as you want to go in fat-reduction, because the fat-free cheeses tend to be rubbery and tasteless.

➡ **Fat-free plain yogurt.**

The fruit yogurts are adulterated dreadfully with sugar. It's enough to make their calorie content soar from about 90 calories per cup to about 250. That is about 10 teaspoons of sugar per cup. Vanilla, coffee, and lemon yogurts are little better. You'll get more flavor and better taste by starting with plain yogurt and adding a teaspoon or two of granulated fructose or honey and a teaspoon or two of an all-fruit spread such as Polaner's. A quarter teaspoon of decaffeinated coffee granules adds plenty of flavor, too.

➡ **Fat-free cottage cheese.**

The dry type keeps better but needs to be cut with plain yogurt or sour cream to be palatably moist when uncooked in or on a dish.

➡ **Fat-free mozzarella cheese.**

➡ **Fat-free cream cheese, Philadelphia Brand or Alpine Lace.**

➡ **Low-fat cheeses.**

As mentioned above, fatless cheeses tend to be tasteless cheeses. A few fatless swisses and mozzarellas, notably Alpine Lace, are okay for eating plain or grating on pasta dishes, but they do not bake well atop an open-face sandwich or pizza. They dry badly and brown to a leatherlike consistency. Part-skim fat-reduced cheeses can taste just as good as their full-fat cousins.

Watch the fat content, realizing that whole-milk cheeses vary from 20 to 60 percent fat and that the fat in cheese is the bad, highly saturated kind. The more translucent the cheese, the more fat in it (not counting the holes in Swiss). Also, the more liquid the cheese, the higher the fat content. Just remember "Brie/ puts fat/ on me." With almost 80 percent butterfat, brie is best thought of nutritionally as semisolid butter.

➠ **Fat-free sour cream.**

Breakstone, Land O Lakes, or house brand only if it has milk solids added (too thin and runny otherwise, or stiffened with gelatin, i.e., the pits).

$\mathcal{O}$ILS, NUTS, SEEDS, SAUCES, VINEGARS

➠ **Expeller-pressed canola oil (plain-tasting).**

➠ **Expeller-pressed walnut oil (sweet-tasting).**

➠ **Expeller-pressed olive oil (tart-tasting).**

Please make a trip to your local health food store and get Hain or another brand of oils that are cold-pressed. Keep them in the cold, dark fridge to preserve the essential fatty acids (see Chapter 8). All the seeds and nuts listed below should be stored in an airless, sealed container in the refrigerator to keep their essential oils from turning rancid.

➠ **Pepitas.**

➠ **Green, unroasted plain pumpkin seeds.**

One of the highest-recommended sources of essential fatty acids. Fine on salads or plain.

➠ **Sesame seeds.**

Roasted, they add nutty taste to bread crusts and salads without adding much fat because they're so tiny.

➠ **Walnuts or almonds.**

Unroasted, they rival pepitas as the best dietary sources of essential fatty acids and have been found to be associated with dramatically lower rates of heart attacks when eaten five or more times weekly. Walnut pieces are cheaper than whole nutmeats, and walnuts are always broken in the recipes in this book.

➠ **Promise Ultra Fat-Free margarine.**

➠ **I Can't Believe It's Not Butter! Spray.**

➠ **Hellman's Fat-Free Mayonnaise.**

➠ **Rice wine vinegar.**

➠ **Tarragon-flavored white vinegar.**

➠ **Apple cider vinegar.**

➠ **Any balsamic red wine vinegar from Modena, Italy.**

Don't neglect these stock items. It's ridiculously easy to make your own salad dressings if you keep good vinegars, plain yogurt, oils, and dried herbs and spices. Mayo, even the fat-free kind, is good for making the dressings creamy (emulsified) instead of separated into two layers. Homemade dressings taste much better than store-bought, and guests will think you're a super-chef when you make them.

𝓕RUITS AND VEGETABLES

FRUITS

Buy at least four kinds of fresh fruits that you like. This is about the minimum for making an interesting fruit salad, which, thanks to my wife, adds great taste and flair to our family's dinners. Think about when you plan to eat your fruit before you buy it. Some fruits have only a one-day shelf life, such as ripe bananas. Some may have a shelf-life of up to two weeks, such as firm apples.

It's discouraging to see fruit go bad. Better to buy too little fresh fruit, enjoy it, and want to return to the grocery to buy more. Buy some canned too, so that you have variety. Get one kind per can, not canned fruit salad, because the flavors always gets homogenized in canned fruit salad. Get fruit that is canned in its own juice if possible. It has the most flavor and the least sugar.

Frozen fruits are a compromise. Freezing and thawing invariably bursts plant cell walls, so thawed frozen fruit is mushy. But it has more taste than canned fruit.

VEGETABLES

Buy at least four kinds of fresh vegetables that you like. [See "Cooking Chinese" for some selections on variety by taste.]

Don't buy the prepackaged, precut fresh vegetable mixes, inviting as they are, unless you plan to cook them before they are outdated and unless your grocer keeps them refrigerated. The outdates on these products are really serious: They go bad quickly after they are washed and cut. They absolutely must be refrigerated in the grocer's, or they're a health menace.

Try each of the following:

➡ **Green onions, bulb onions (half-grown white onions that look like overgrown green onions), Vidalia onions, or Texas sweet onions.**

Don't be afraid. The recipes make these things tolerable, even for the stomach-impaired.

➡ **Russet potatoes, Idahos if available.**

As with fruits, buy for the short term. Unrefrigerated potatoes get soft and start growing in a couple of weeks. Refrigerated potatoes can take up a lot of room, and they shed dirt, and they get soft and rot.

Unless you're cooking for more than two people, be a sport and buy potatoes individually. You can restrict your choices to potatoes that haven't been hacked or bludgeoned. They don't rot on the outside unless you mistreat them. They store longer, and they won't surprise you with rotten interiors.

➡ **Beans, lentils, etc.**

First, keep dry versions for when you have time to cook them. Lentils and split peas cook the fastest, in as little as 30 to 45 minutes. Great northern or navy beans are the blandest, which means they take to other flavors the most easily.

Black beans and garbanzos are the most difficult to digest and the tastiest.

Kidney beans and red beans are intermediate in taste and digestibility.

All dry beans keep well at room temperature. They should be kept in airtight containers to keep out pests. Keep them dry so they don't sprout. There's no stigma attached to using canned beans. There may be a great amount of sodium, and there may be a lot of saturated fat added, as in most (but not all) brands of refried beans, so read labels before buying.

GRAINS AND CEREALS

RICE

➡ **Brown, long-grain white, and wild rice.**

You may like basmati rice better than white rice, as it is a bit more nutty-tasting. A blend of stronger-tasting brown rices such as Lundberg's may please you even more than wild rice, which is not really a rice at all.

➡ **Medium-grain rice.**

This is essential if you want to make risotto. It leaks some of its interior out into the liquid in which it cooks, making a gravy for itself.

FLOUR AND OTHER GRAIN PRODUCTS

➡ **Unbleached bread flour or all-purpose unbleached white flour.**

➡ **Whole wheat flour.**

Turns rancid at room temperature. Store in refrigerator for less than 6 months.

➡ **Oats, quick-cooking (1 minute) rolled oats.**

These are the most versatile, and they are identical to the long-cooking kind except for being squashed flatter. They can be used for cookies, muffins, crumb toppings, even thickening sauces, as well as for cereal.

⇒ **Wheat berries.**

A.k.a. bulgur or bulgur wheat, used to make tabbouli or zestier pancakes.

⇒ **Oat bran flour, Hodgson Mills.**

This is not all oat bran; it's wheat flour with a percentage of oat bran in it.

⇒ **Pasta shapes.**

Keep some ready-made pasta for those times when you don't feel like making pasta for yourself. Get the dry stuff, not the wet stuff from the refrigerators in the dairy section of the supermarket, so it's always handy and doesn't deteriorate.

Keep a few varieties in addition to spaghetti, including pastas that cook very fast, such as angel hair and couscous. This lets you add good stuff to thin soups quickly. It also lets you get suppers to the table fast. Orzo, rice-shaped pasta, helps you avoid panic when you are making a stir fry and find the cupboard bare of rice.

⇒ **Ready-to-eat breakfast cereals.**

Get a few simple kinds that give you whole-grain taste and let you add sweeteners for yourself. Old favorites such as Cheerios, shredded wheat, and corn flakes have now been joined by exotics like puffed kashi. Avoid the pre-sweetened cereals (read the labels). Otherwise you wind up with a breakfast food that is at least one-third sugar.

Don't buy high-fiber breakfast cereals as a substitute for eating plenty of fiber in every meal. If you still need bran to move your bowels, fine—buy a breakfast cereal with bran. Again, read labels and compare. Some bran cereals have more bran than others. The labels will also help you avoid getting stuck with a load of sugar.

Don't eat a wheat bran cereal to lower your cholesterol, either. Wheat bran is an insoluble type that does not bind cholesterol and thus does not lower the levels of cholesterol in the blood. Oat bran does that; rice bran does that; wheat bran does not.

Snacking

This is a section about munching. We're talking *raiding* here, not cooking. You know, opening the refrigerator or pantry cabinet, pulling out goodies, and eating them as they are. Recently, this may often have helped your hunger pains, only to induce stomach pains later. *This can become pure fun again for you.*

Plan ahead and stock up. Late at night, you can either comfort your stomach or make it miserable. It's your choice!

BREADS

It's hard to beat bread for a ready-to-eat snack. Whole-grain breads give more chewing satisfaction and take longer to digest, so they last longer. Pita and foccacia give the most chewing satisfaction, because they are the crustiest.

The problem for the stomach and for the heart is not the bread but the toppings that make it wetter and more satisfying. (See the bread-spread recipe in Chapter 14 for a good start on making bread appetizing.)

In the next section, you'll find a selection of high-protein toppings. Don't forget the cool, sweet, or tangy veggies to go on bread, too. Try romaine rather than iceberg lettuce to get some nutrition instead of 97 percent water. See if you tolerate tomato by the fresh slice even if you don't tolerate tomato products when concentrated in sauces or pastes.

HIGH-PROTEIN SNACKS

Spreads, dips, sandwich fillings—there are lots of different high-protein snacks to help keep you from feeling hungry for the rest of the night. Thin-sliced turkey ham gives a lot of satisfaction per amount consumed. It can be quite salty, so use it to add flavor to snacks rather than filling up on it.

If you experiment with fat-free and low-fat cheeses, you may give up on the fat-free kinds. They are pretty rubbery. Alpine Lace Swiss cheese and mozzarella are the only fatless cheeses I finish when I bring such things home.

Fat-free sour cream is a comforting spread or dip, adding cool richness. It's about lactose-free, so lactose-intolerant people can indulge in it. Fat-free cream cheese is good with crackers.

Fat-free cottage cheese has all the taste of regular cottage cheese, but it does lack the creaminess. First try it on a dish where it plays second fiddle. Fresh (rather than canned) fruit does it good. Top with low-fat or fat-free grated parmesan if it must be the main flavor. Weight Watchers grated parmesan is an excellent helper.

Soy links, veggie burgers, and hot-dogs are high in protein and either fat-free or low-fat (read the labels). They are included here because some people like such things cold rather than hot. (No, I won't sink to including cold slices of pizza here.)

All-fruit jams will match or exceed the glycemic index of the fruit for which they are named, because they tend to have a high amount of sugar from grape juice concentrate. Use them sparingly.

If you can get your hands on home-smoked fish, you can avoid excessive quantities of salt. That is about the only way known to me to enjoy reasonably healthy smoked fish. Smoked soy "cheese" can add relish to sandwiches and pizzas, but the taste isn't so hot that I'd eat it by itself.

A bit of thin-sliced raw tuna or salmon is fashionable not only in Japan but throughout the U.S. now, of course. Inspection of fish being what it is in this country, it would not be prudent to try this at home from fresh fish. An exception could be made if you have a reliable fish market, keep your fresh fish on ice (not just in the refrigerator), and use it within 24 hours of purchase. Check with the person behind the counter at the fish market before you try this.

People in the far north, white and Eskimo alike, swear by eating raw fish while it is still frozen. Crunchy sushi doesn't appeal to me, though.

Cold beans? How about baba ganoush? This spread, made from garbanzos, is yummy on pita bread. If you get it from the deli, ask first if it has ingredients that offend your stomach. One of our favorite delis has baba ganoush with or without garlic.

CRUNCHY CARBOHYDRATE SNACKS

Louise's Potato Chips have a negligible amount of fat, officially zero grams of fat and zero calories from fat per 1-ounce serving. Baked, these chips are every bit as crunchy as regular potato chips, which have up to 40 percent of calories as fat. They feel more brittle and sharper in the mouth than regular potato chips. Chew them a little slower so you don't poke your mouth. They accept dips well, but get soggy fast in a humid atmosphere or in casseroles.

Louise's, Guiltless Gourmet, and even Frito Lays now make corn chips that are virtually fat-free (whole-corn chips can't be fat-free, since corn contains corn oil). These chips are not as crunchy as fried tortilla chips. They're okay with fat-free sour cream or a mild bean dip. If they make you miss fried corn chips, as happens to me, that does you a disservice.

SnackWells pepper crackers sit well in my stomach, and their wheat crackers do too. The various health food store crackers such as Health Valley lack salt as well as fat. This makes them low-taste, but you can do something about that if you keep sliced turkey ham handy. Eating them with fat-free cream cheese is another worthwhile option.

Pretzels are low-fat, though they may have huge amounts of salt. Have you tried oat bran pretzels? Penny Sticks makes a pretzel nugget that is tasty, very low-fat at 1 gram per 1-ounce serving, and has "only" 110 milligrams of sodium per ounce. It's just salty enough to have some taste. A friend of mine tried them, said, "Tastes like cardboard," and reached for more. When I challenged him about this, he said, "But I *like* cardboard."

Breadsticks cut out the salt as well as the fat and give a good crunch. Pick a brand with whole wheat as the first ingredient if you can find one, because plain white bread sticks are so full of air that they tend to be all crunch, no taste. Sesame seeds add plenty of taste, too. Try dipping them in breadspread (see Chapter 14) or your favorite all-fruit jam.

Rice cakes are worth a try also, but don't assume all are fat-free or low-salt. Read the labels. Don't try these without having something to drink handy, as they seem extraordinarily dry and can stick in the throats of people with esophageal disorders.

Mad at the national biscuit-makers for their exaggerated claims of "low-fat" in their crackers? Try munching Chex cereals or a shredded wheat biscuit (without milk) instead of crackers.

Chex take to other flavors well, and you don't have to drown them in garlic to make a tasty, crunchy party mix. Shredded wheat is messy to eat dry, but it's yummy with a little salt or NuSalt.

FRUITS AND VEGETABLES

One of the great things about fruits and many vegetables is how ready to eat they are. Their Achilles' heel is their short shelf life. Don't be too much of a snob to keep frozen vegetables and canned fruits on hand.

Vegetables are generally blanched before they are frozen. Opening the package, pouring the contents into a strainer, and running the vegetable under water for a few seconds may be enough to thaw it and make it quite palatable, depending on your taste.

Plain and semi-crunchy vegetables can be good. Dipped in a favorite dip or salad dressing (see Chapter 16), they can be yummy. A few frozen veggies, such as peas, can be poured out of the frozen container and eaten as is, especially in a mix of other (not-so-cold) items.

The fruits that are canned in their own juices (or some other mild fruit juice) instead of in syrup taste best. Especially recommended: Dole Tropical Fruit Salad, Mott's chunky apple sauces without sugar, and any brand of pineapple in its own juice.

Now, don't think I'm nuts, but my highest recommendation among canned fruit is Gerber's (or other) baby food strained fruits. Extra-good because of the focus on quality rather than quantity, these foods are sensational as a snack for one, either plain in their handy little containers, or stirred into some plain yogurt.

DAIRY GOODS AND IMITATORS

Cheeses and sour creams were discussed already. Milk can be very satisfying and refreshing, especially with some of the new fat-free or low-fat cookies such as Frookies and SnackWells.

If you like milk but have learned to avoid its high content of saturated fat, don't kid yourself by using 2 percent milk and thinking you are doing your arteries a favor. Go to 1 percent milk. By the end of a quart, it will probably taste all right to you. Then start mixing it 50–50 with skim milk. If this too is okay by the end of a quart, go all the way to skim.

If you dislike skim milk for its thinness, try mixing a tablespoon or two of dry milk per quart of skim milk. An alternative is Lactaid or another brand of lactose-reduced milk, which has more taste even if it is skim.

Weight Watchers makes the best-tasting skim milk powder I've found. It is not yellow or burnt-tasting. Individual packets of it last indefinitely and are very handy for adding to drinks or cereal.

Up to 70 percent of the adult population is lactose-intolerant. This means we can't digest the high levels of lactose in cow's milk. It goes on undigested to the large intestine, where it is fermented to gas or even produces diarrhea one to five hours after having milk or milk products.

Lactose-intolerant people may feel fine after drinking lactose-reduced milk. Supermarket dairy cases stock milk that is 70 percent lactose-reduced. Lactaid has also introduced a 100 percent lactose-free milk. These milks have nothing removed, only an enzyme added that has broken down the lactose to galactose and glucose. This makes the milk taste somewhat sweeter, but it's not exactly a fountain treat.

If you don't like this level of sweetness, you can buy pills of the enzyme as Lactaid (or other brands). The enzyme in the pill breaks down the lactose if you take it just before drinking regular milk.

Soy or rice "milk" is available in health food stores and even in some supermarkets. It has a long shelf life, even after opened, if kept refrigerated. The soy version has a distinct taste of a grain to many people.

Try the rice version first. It is closer to cow's milk. A vanilla-flavored version is available, and may be preferable with cold cereal.

Imitation cheeses are sky-high in salt content. They also may be sky-high in fat content. Read the labels before buying. They are not recommended because they are synthetic.

Chapter 13

REFRESHING BEVERAGES

First, I offer a review to remind you of the beverages to avoid so your stomach won't make you suffer. Then I list some decent hot drinks you can get at the supermarket, and some exotic brews.

HOT DRINKS

NO-NO #1: COFFEE, AND SUBSTITUTES FOR IT

Caffeine and Coffee Addiction. Fresh-brewed coffee is highest in caffeine, with 90 to 120 milligrams (per 6- to 8-ounce cup). The sugared and flavored instants are lowest, with no more than 60 milligrams. All coffees except decaffeinated are higher in caffeine than tea, which has 30 to 60 milligrams. Colas and some other sodas are caffeinated, of course, with 30 to almost 60 milligrams of caffeine per cup.

Drink these beverages every day for months or years and you are likely to be addicted. If you cannot think clearly in the morning after a decent night's sleep until you have a cup of coffee, you are addicted. That is, you are suffering from a *withdrawal syndrome to caffeine* that you are medicating with that first cup of the morning. *Addicted* doesn't just mean slavishly keen on the effects of a drug. It means several things, one of which is spending considerable effort to secure a supply of the drug to prevent withdrawal effects.

The brain accommodates the stimulant effect of caffeine by shutting down its synthesis of its own chemicals that act in the same way. You know how this works if you have learned to stop drinking coffee in the afternoon or early evening so that you can sleep at night. The caffeine lasts for about 4 to 6 hours, then it is lost to the brain. The brain doesn't switch on its synthesis of alerting chemicals for days after this. In between time, the addict easily falls asleep. But he or she cannot become alert again the next morning without a new supply of caffeine.

Caffeine also acts as a nasal decongestant, so the addict who stops drinking coffee may get a raging sinus headache and blocked nasal passages for a few days.

Like any addiction, there are two main ways of breaking caffeine addiction. One is to go "cold turkey." After three days or so, one wakes up better and the headache clears.

The other approach is to cut back slowly. Anywhere along the line between full-bore caffeine use and no caffeine use, one can declare stability and stop trying to cut back farther. You can decide when the level of use and the symptoms are comfortable. Switching to tea or half-decaf can help in doing this.

Decaffeinated Coffee. Decaffeinated coffee is virtually the same as whole coffee, except for the caffeine. It has as much as 97 percent of the caffeine removed, but that's about all. The manufacturers have gone as far as they can to make it simulate whole coffee. The same wake-up aroma, the same great bitter taste, the same sexy couples in the TV commercials.

Don't let this fool you. If you have stomach problems, don't substitute decaffeinated coffee for regular coffee in an attempt to stop the stomach irritation that coffee causes. It won't work. It's not the caffeine that irritates the stomach, it's the rest of what is in coffee.

Coffee is acidic. This irritates the stomach directly. Coffee also stimulates acid secretion by the stomach lining. This makes it irritate the stomach more. In people with normal stomachs, this effect lasts for less than an hour. However, in people with stomach trouble, everything that causes distress seems to last longer, including the irritant effects of coffee.

Tea and Maté. Tea, especially Japanese green tea, is now touted as a great substitute for coffee. Tea is high in potassium, for one thing. It may have other good effects, too, warding off the chronic diseases of aging.

Regular tea tastes somewhat sweet, especially orange pekoe. This is what coffee drinkers have against it, I think. They want a jolt not only of caffeine but also of bitterness, or bitterness balanced by milk with sweetness and creaminess for a more complex taste.

Anyone determined to switch over should try English (or Irish) Breakfast, a black tea that is much less sweet and much more bitter. It stands up to milk, keeping its character without turning into warm, slightly discolored milk. Tea made the English way, strong enough to look black, is definitely higher in caffeine. A 30-second brew has about 30 milligrams of caffeine; a 5-minute brew has about 60.

Tea is high in compounds called tannins. Tannins are good applied locally for soothing, for example, for sunburned skin, but they add a dry taste to tea. Tannins are used to make leather out of animal hide. This should be enough to tell you how dry they can make your mouth.

Green tea has a grassy taste that you may or may not like. It is not sweet at all. It's very refreshing drunk hot with food, especially salty food.

Maté is a Brazilian beverage that is sometimes substituted wholly for coffee and sometimes added to it or to tea. It has caffeine in it, but is not known to irritate the stomach. It hasn't bothered me when I've tried it, but I don't know of any medical effects from it.

Herb Tea. So many herb teas are available nowadays that it's practically impossible not to find one you like.

Want fruity? You've got it: Celestial Seasonings, Bigelow, and Lipton's are at your service in a bunch of flavors each. Add a teaspoon of honey to round out the fruitiness if you wish. Start with orange-flavored teas, the oldest stand-bys. Raspberry and blackberry are also quite fruity. Strawberry and some others can be a bit limp unless you use only half a cup of water per teabag, because the original taste is weaker.

Want tart? Try Red Zinger or Lemon Zinger from Celestial. Their sourness stands up to being iced. These teas are so sour that you may want to dilute them by using more than a cup of water per bag.

Want dessert-y? Try Yogi cinnamon or vanilla with milk, or try the mixes that The Nature Company sells. These loose-tea mixes are heavenly, some so sweet that sugar is not needed. Another very dessert-y sweet tea is the licorice-flavored herb tea from Stash.

Want earthy or bitter, like coffee? Try Native American teas. Well brewed, they stand up to milk almost as well as English Breakfast tea does.

Also try decaffeinated teas. Decaf tea mixtures enlarge the taste compared to pure infusions. The fruit teas get more sweetness and body from the mixture with real tea, even if the tea taste is diluted somewhat by the decaffeinating process. Bigelow's Cinnamon Stick and Constant Comment are available decaffeinated.

No-No's #2 and #3: Cocoa and Minty Teas

Cocoa seems to be a pure comfort food. It won't keep you up unless you are unusually sensitive, because it has only a tad of caffeine-like substances in it. However, it directly relaxes the lower esophageal sphincter, so it contributes to esophageal reflux. You may find that the milk you mix it with prevents this effect.

To make cocoa, don't follow the package directions. Use half a teaspoon or, at most, a level teaspoon of dry cocoa rather than more. It will need much less sugar (whoops, I mean granulated fructose) to balance the bitter taste.

Make the flavor of cocoa more dessert-y with a teaspoon of vanilla and a sprinkle of cinnamon. Stir the cocoa, fructose, vanilla, and cinnamon with just a tablespoon of hot water at first, to disperse the cocoa well. Then add hot water to fill your cup three-quarters full. Then add milk. This avoids having to heat the milk, which scalds it into scum all too easily.

Mint also reduces lower esophageal sphincter pressure. It is present in all the old antacids for this very reason. It helps anyone with simple indigestion and heartburn to burp up the carbon dioxide that is formed when the antacid neutralizes stomach acid.

The trouble is, people with esophageal reflux don't need their LES pressure to be lower; they need it higher, to keep the acidic stomach contents from rising up and burning the esophagus.

Mint is a frequent component of herb teas. Chamomile teas such as Sleepy Time and Moonlight Mint have varying levels of mint. Sleepy Time is about the lightest in mint of these mixes. If you get nighttime reflux after drinking one of these teas, assume that mint is the culprit and stop drinking it.

Plain chamomile tea has sweetness and fruitiness. It does need a full 5 minutes of brewing to develop a rich, golden color and satisfying taste.

COLD DRINKS

NO-NO #1: ALCOHOL

Alcohol in moderate or low doses helps a rat's stomach. It induces the production in the stomach of cytoprotective prostaglandins. These chemicals help a rat avoid ulcers when exposed to drugs that cause ulcers. The stomach secretes its own version of Cytotec®, the prostaglandin drug that helps the stomachs of people taking anti-inflammatory drugs for arthritis.

I wouldn't doubt that the same thing happens to normal people chronically exposed to hot peppers and other stomach irritants. People who get ulcers, esophageal reflux and heartburn, or plain old indigestion are not lab rats. Alcohol hurts our stomach linings.

I tried to find how low a dose of red wine I could take to get its beneficial effects for the heart. There was none. Even half a small glass of red wine bothered my stomach, and even when I took it with a bland dinner. If you want to try this, start small, with just an ounce or two of wine, and have it with, not before, a bland dinner. Don't be surprised if, like me, you find there is no dose that is safe for your stomach. That is why alcohol in all forms is to be eliminated in all the diets for stomach disease.

Alcohol in low doses does two contrary things to the brain: It stimulates and it depresses. The stimulant effect comes first, before the concentrations rise much. This is why some drinkers are convivial, even boisterous. Then, with higher concentrations, alcohol depresses brain and nerve function. Even this produces contradictory effects, because depressing some excitatory functions of the brain allays anxiety, as with shy people who blossom at parties only after drinking.

Alcohol is a temporary "cure" for social phobia or even panic disorder. It also may suppress excitability beyond a certain point, which is why alcohol classically makes men impotent. It slows reaction time, of course, and impairs judgment, why is why alcohol and driving don't mix.

In our society, taking advantage of the enjoyable aspects of alcohol is socially acceptable. It is even encouraged. This adds to the difficulty in saying "No" to an alcoholic drink at a party or from a partner or friend who wants us to let our inhibitions down or just relax.

Nowadays, fortunately, this is easing, for several reasons. We drive everywhere, and even the brewers and winegrowers include cautionary words in their ads because alcohol causes so much mayhem on the highway. Also, alcohol deforms the fetus, and the government has gotten into the act, requiring warnings to women.

Not drinking alcohol is also becoming fashionable because of the growing movement not to harm oneself with any sort of chemicals. Alcohol is not a natural component of food. It is a chemical, the original psychoactive chemical, handed down to us for thousands of years. Only fermentation produces it, a process induced by microorganisms acting on sugar in fruit or grain.

Eating or drinking things that have been changed utterly by microorganisms is not ordinarily a safe act. Drinking alcohol in quantities that affect our brains is not a safe act.

If you miss the taste of beer, try the nonalcoholic types. If you miss the taste of wine, your loss is the greater, for the nonalcoholic wines are not very comparable to the real thing. You may find fruit beverages an acceptable substitute. A few suggestions follow.

FRUIT BEVERAGES

Fruit drinks have gone through a great resurgence in the last ten years or so. For the younger set who want something as sweet as soda pop but without the fizz, there are plenty of fruit-flavored drinks. These are unlikely to appeal to adults because they are so high in sugar. This makes them yet another strain on the blood sugar–insulin system discussed in the chapter on carbohydrates.

Some fruit beverages include carbonation to help balance the sweetness, so don't just go by taste. Read the label to find out if a drink can send your blood sugar into orbit and then make it crash.

More refreshing alone or with a meal are the all-fruit drinks. A couple of brands of real, all-fruit beverages stand out in quality and taste: R. W. Knudsen and After the Fall. As with wines, delicate, less-sweet fruit drinks go better with delicate-tasting lunches and dinners. Some, such as peach-flavored and berry-flavored drinks, are so fruity that cutting them one-to-one with ice water works well.

You'll find that sourness hangs on better than sweetness does in diluted drinks. Another tasty way to bring the balance of tastes to tartness is to add a slug of orange or cranberry juice (not cranberry cocktails, which are mostly sugars and water). This makes the juices less tolerable to sensitive stomachs, though.

Try Concord grape juice with pizza; cherry fruit drink with Chinese food; peach or diluted berry drinks with chicken dishes; white grape juice with vegetarian meals.

Apple cider appeals to all. Nutritionally, it must be recognized as virtually nothing but sugar, albeit natural sugar, and water. Watch out for the ones "from concentrate," as they tend to carry the same bitter taste as bruised "grounder" apples.

The carbonated ciders such as Martinelli's tend to be so full-bodied that you may drink less of them, which is one way of saving on sugar intake. The way they are put up in bottles like champagne helps give their use a festive air.

Citrus beverages are not a good idea for the digestively impaired. I do so much better off them completely that it's worth the trade-off to me. You may try to determine your own tolerance for them, if you wish. They're so tasty that it's hard to give them up entirely.

You may find that a dab of orange, grapefruit, or lemon in something else gives you the tartness and enjoyment that you want. Try adding the citrus to plain, sparkling water. Dress it up with a twist of lemon or lime or with a chunk of pineapple or a small wedge of a sweet orange. Or try adding an ounce of orange or grapefruit juice to a beverage that is a little too sweet, maybe a peach juice drink.

ICED TEAS

Iced tea is refreshing in hot weather. Do not forget that it contains caffeine, however. A friend of mine drank it all the day and then couldn't understand why she didn't sleep at night. The sweetness of tea makes it more palatable as a cold beverage for many people.

Decaffeinated tea works for iced tea, but you have to use plenty of it. One bag makes no more than a small cupful of tea, because the decaffeination process usually uses water, and that extracts a lot of the flavor. So for a big 12-ounce glass of iced tea, you may have to use two or more decaffeinated tea bags to get a flavor that isn't too thin after it's chilled and diluted with ice.

There are plenty of tea substitutes without caffeine available. See the section on herb teas, under hot beverages. Some herb teas are made especially to be iced. The Iced Delight series from Celestial Seasonings is one group. These sweeter, browner teas hold up to icing quite well.

No-No #2: Soda Pop, Regular and Diet

I've already included a diatribe against sugar-sweetened soda, in Chapter 7. To add to that, carbonation is bad for those of us with susceptible stomachs. It's acid, and the pressure it causes makes the lower esophageal sphincter fly open, spilling acid back into the esophagus where it can injure the tissues.

Then there is the issue of the so-called diet sodas. Why do people order a large cheeseburger, fries, and a diet soda? This makes absolutely no sense to me. If you're going to inflict 60 grams of fat on yourself, why not go for the gusto and get real sugar in your soda pop? How much more harm could it do you?

Ah, but I'm not in tune with advertising. The ads for the fast-food restaurants show people who are not overweight enjoying themselves on the cheeseburgers and fries, typically young adults with happy children. The ads for the "diet" sodas show sleek, slender people. Put them together, and what have you got? Enjoyment and slimming!

No, what you've really got is advertising fertilizer. At minimum, people have a tendency toward self-delusion when they're drinking diet beverages. Consciously or unconsciously, the idea is that if you're having a diet drink, you can eat much more food than you normally would.

This is the minimum harm done. We do not know the long-term effects on health of ingesting artificial sweeteners. We know the long-term effects on laboratory animals, but we do not know the effects on humans, especially juveniles.

Cold Drinks for Parties or Other Special Enjoyments

Smoothies are combinations of fruit, milk, and ice, mixed together in a blender until—guess what?—smooth. It's hard to go wrong with these three kinds of ingredients. Keep the amount of fruit up and the amount of ice down (no more than about four cubes per cup), or else you get a beverage that is too watery. Chill the fruit beforehand or the smoothie won't be cold enough.

Using a banana per cupful of smoothie gives a lot of taste and body. A little mango goes a long way. Seedy fruit will leave a heavy residue on the bottom, but who cares? Don't expect the blender to do anything with pits except dull itself. Remember that some pits, for example, wild cherry, are poisonous. If you use berries, you may have to add honey or apple juice to the mix.

Honey is hard to mix into cold beverages, as it congeals in the cold, so mash it with the fruit before adding it to the main mix. Granulated fructose dissolves well in the blender. It is quite sweet, but can be used just as you would regular sugar in ice-chilled smoothies, because its super-sweetness is not appreciable in the cold.

Cinnamon goes with nearly every fruited thing, so try it mixed in or dashed on top. Nutmeg is much more tart and complex. If you use it, sprinkle just a dusting on top or it takes over.

Punch is a mixture that usually has some sherbet or sorbet, fruit juice, and a little carbonation in it. Contrary to your memories, you can make punch that is refreshing and neither icky-sweet nor alcoholic.

Use a cup of your favorite juices, skip the carbonated beverage, and stir in a quarter to half a cup of a fruity flavor of sorbet or frozen yogurt that you like. Keep it in a chilled or insulated container until it is served.

Shakes and Sodas do not require ice cream. Nonfat ice milk or frozen yogurt shakes can be delicious. Blend them with good flavors so they will delight rather than disappoint.

For a chocolate shake, dissolve half a teaspoon of real cocoa, a teaspoon of granulated fructose, and a pinch of cinnamon in a tablespoon of hot water. Mix with a spoon. Then add the milk and ice milk or frozen yogurt.

For a strawberry shake, use a quarter of a cup of berries. Mash them with a teaspoon of granulated fructose or brown sugar. Add milk and ice milk or frozen yogurt.

For a vanilla shake, add a whole teaspoon of vanilla extract and a dash of cinnamon.

Want a root beer float? Use Hires, IBC, Dad's, A & W, or another full-bodied root beer rather than a synthetic concoction like Fanta.

Water is always fashionable. How to pick a water? By your taste only. Avoid the ones with lots of carbonation, or else pour them from the height of your extended arm into an unchilled glass. Done with a flourish, this looks elegant and drives most of the carbonation out.

Chapter 14

WHAT'S FOR BREAKFAST?

In America, breakfast tends to be packed with grease, sugar, or both. A plate of eggs with sausage or bacon and hash browns just doesn't cut it anymore for those who want their hearts to age no more rapidly than the rest of them does.

Toaster pastries and sweetened cereals make your blood glucose rocket up and down again so fast that it can make your head swim, literally, and make you fat (see Chapter 7). Donuts and coffee don't even begin to give you complete nutrition.

But you don't have to sit down to a platter of grease to get a hearty breakfast, nor let yourself stay trained to believe that breakfast equals sugar, even in this country of instant everything.

A 400-calorie, energy-packed way to start the day is with a cup of whole-grain cereal such as oatmeal, with skim milk and a banana or a handful of raisins for sweetness, plus two slices of whole-grain toast with breadspread (see next section) or a fruit butter. It's quick, and it will perk up your brainpower for the morning.

If you want more warmth and solidity, scramble a carton of egg substitute and add an ounce of strips of either turkey Canadian bacon or ham. Have a glass of a non-citrus juice with it, so you get your vitamins and minerals without too much acid.

You want something more exotic? Some of the recipes in this chapter are a little off the beaten path, but they are all hearty and nutritious.

In any case, go for a balanced breakfast—one with enough carbohydrates for energy, enough protein to sustain you for the morning, and some fruit to supply vitamins, minerals, and good flavor.

Getting enough protein is a must. Otherwise, blood sugar ebbs again in a couple of hours and one can get tired, fuzzy-headed, or irritable. How much is enough protein? Aim for 10 grams. Two ounces of cold cereal provides about 6 grams of not-so-great-quality protein. To this high-carbohydrate (about 50 grams) start for a meal, add a source of high-quality protein: half a cup of skim milk has 4 grams; a cup of soy milk has 3 to 7.

Half a cup of plain nonfat or low-fat yogurt has 6 grams of protein. Just watch out for the commercially sweetened ones. They sugar up the carbo count to 43 grams per cup! A generous teaspoonful of honey or brown sugar (about 5 grams of sugar) on top of half a cup of yogurt may very well be all the sugar you'd want.

Better still, skip all the sugar and add high-quality protein in solid form. A single ounce of lean smoked turkey Canadian bacon or ham has 9 to 10 grams of protein. An ounce of tempeh or 3 ounces of extra-firm tofu has the same. A slice of low-fat cheese (part-skim mozzarella or low-fat Swiss) or soy cheese (1 ounce) has 6 to 8 grams of good-quality protein.

For fruit, you can't beat blueberries. These sweet-tart morsels are right up there with broccoli in providing wonderful antioxidants. Strawberries (organic, please) are also good providers.

Grapes, apples, and bananas are other good low-acid fruit choices for people with dyspepsia. Avoid citrus and pineapple except as garnishes because of their high acid content. A tangerine, some Mandarin orange wedges, or their little Spanish cousins the clementines are wonderfully sweet, small, and may have a low enough amount of acid for you to tolerate if you can resist having more than one.

ℬREADSPREAD

What's breakfast without butter? Muffins, butter, and jam. Waffles or pancakes, butter and syrup. Hot, buttered toast. A pat of butter on hot oatmeal. Hash browns with butter on top.

Then came The Diet. Sugar-free fruit butter was the only spread allowed. Oatmeal was supposed to be plain except for maybe some raisins or a banana. Hash browns? Forget it!

I missed butter a lot. Butter is essentially all fat, and the worst kinds. In it, what isn't ordinary saturated fatty acid is trans-fatty acid! But it tastes unique, a little sweetness from the glycerol, a little tang like mild cheese, and a buttery feel from short-chain, easy-melting, water-soluble fats. It gets into the tongue to the taste buds instead of just coating it greasily as long-chain fats in margarine do. Your taste buds require any food to dissolve before you can taste it, so butter has more taste than margarine.

Oh yeah, sure, you can taste margarine, too. They put enough salt and milk solids in it to give it some flavor. But let's face it, those are different flavors than butter has.

When I developed heart trouble and GERD, I cut out the butter. Eventually I even got over wanting the taste of butter on baked potatoes. On my hot, fresh, homemade muffins. On freshly steamed green beans. On homemade cinnamon raisin bread, warm and soft, fresh from my bread-baker. On boiled sweet corn. . . . Who am I trying to kid? If you grew up with butter, you're going to miss it.

Oh, I tried substitutes.

Fat-free cream cheese is okay on something as substantial as a bagel. But a bagel is that rare starchy food that is as tough as fat-free cream cheese, so it's a fair fight for attention in your mouth.

Fat-free margarine seemed like a wonderful find in the grocery store, before I tried it. It moistens toast okay, but the taste is not even on the same planet as butter. Really, it tastes like it's synthesized out of neutrons by space aliens. What else could give absolutely no taste resembling earth food?

Then I produced a mixture that actually does it. Makes me want to eat bread again. Makes vegetables appealing. Try it and see if you don't agree. This low-fat buttery spread can be made in about two minutes, so don't be put off by how long the recipe looks.

Ingredient	Amount
Philadelphia brand fat-free cream-cheese	4 ounces (use half an 8-ounce package)
Promise Ultra fat-free margarine	4 ounces (use half an 8-ounce tub)
Canola oil, expeller-pressed, if available	$\frac{1}{4}$ to $\frac{1}{3}$ cup

Start with the ingredients cold if you want, but they mix more easily if they are at room temperature. Take a one-pint round plastic bowl or freezer container with cover. In it, cream (soften by mashing) the cream cheese with a fork. Add about half of the margarine. Mix with a fork till the color's even. Add the rest of the margarine and mix till the color's even and no lumps remain. Add 1/4 cup of oil. Mix carefully a hundred strokes till it stops trying to separate and it thickens. Taste.

If it's buttery-slick enough for your taste, fine. If not, add the rest of the oil and mix until it thickens. Warning: With 1/3 cup of oil, the spread separates easily and must be kept refrigerated. With just 1/4 cup of oil, it may get a little cheesy-tough when refrigerated.

When made with 1/4 cup of oil, this spread has less than 1 g of fat per teaspoon. Of this, close to half is essential fatty acids. Butter or margarine have 4 g of fat per teaspoon and almost no essential fatty acids. The spread is also a significant source of good-quality protein.

Don't pollute your arteries with any oil but fresh, expeller-pressed canola. Get it from the health food store.

The emulsifiers in Promise, labeled as mono- and di-glycerides, have important functions in this recipe. They hold the mix together, keeping it from separating into oil-based and water-based parts, and they add sweetness. They're sweeter than fats, which are triglycerides. In the latter, the sweet glycerol (glycerin) part of the molecule is more surrounded by fatty acids and hidden from your taste buds.

Store breadspread covered and refrigerated. This will help keep the oil emulsified, so the mix looks appetizing. If it's too stiff at refrigerator temperature, microwave for a few seconds, maybe 15. This spread softens fast in the microwave. Or you can soften it by adding more oil, up to equal proportions with either of the two other ingredients.

This spread is good for cooking and for mixing with other foods, as in icing and sauces. If you forget to stick your breadspread back in the fridge, you can remix with a fork, but it may not get entirely smooth. If it smells good, eat it. If it doesn't, compost it.

MUFFINS

The word *muffin*, meaning "a little muff," is apparently derived from that furry or woolly tube people used to wear to keep their hands warm. Homemade muffins can warm your fingers indeed when piping hot from the oven. That's when they taste best, but first let them cool for five minutes or so, rolled in a towel and tucked into a big bowl. This rehydrates the waxed muffin cup liners. Otherwise the muffins will tend to stick in the muffin cup liners too much to be released.

This is one hazard of going low-fat. When we used to use twice as much oil in the recipes, the muffins released from the cup liners easily, even when very hot.

The recipes here are made for the usual 2¼-inch muffin pan. It makes a dozen muffins at a time and is what the waxed muffin cups fit. These little muffins are so easy to handle that it doesn't matter how fall-apart their texture is. Unless the muffins are just a side dish in a bigger meal, allow two to three per eater. When fresh and hot, they go fast.

Nowadays, the commercial version of a muffin is something large, a muffin that's big enough to make a meal all by itself. "Texas Size" Silverstone® pans are easily available to bake them at home too—without the outrageously high fat content of commercial muffins, which may have as much as 30 grams of fat apiece. The pans for home baking have six muffin cups per pan. You can use them for any of the muffin recipes in this section, but the manufacturer recommends that you use them in a 375-degree oven and bake muffins for 25 to 30 minutes.

Wheat Germ Muffins

Ingredient	Amount
White flour	1 cup
Baking powder	1 teaspoon
NuSalt	½ teaspoon
Egg substitute	¼ cup
Canola oil	⅛ cup
Orange marmalade	⅓ cup
Wheat germ	¼ cup
Skim milk	¼ cup
Lemon juice	1 teaspoon
Granulated fructose	3 tablespoons

Blend the first three ingredients in a small bowl. Separately, stir the other ingredients together in a medium-size bowl. Add the blended dry ingredients, and mix together just until moist (not smooth). Make nine regular-size muffins. Put ¼ inch of cool tap water in the rest of the muffin tray so the muffins cook evenly. Bake in a preheated oven at 400° for about 20 minutes, until the muffins brown a little on top.

Wallbanger Muffins

Make wheat germ muffins as above, but add 1 teaspoon rum extract and 1 tablespoon Galliano liqueur before mixing. The alcohol bakes out.

Whole-Grain Cereal Muffins

Ingredient	Amount
White flour	1 ¼ cup
Baking powder	2 teaspoons
NuSalt	½ teaspoon
Egg substitute	¼ cup
Canola oil	⅛ cup
Molasses	2 tablespoons
Skim milk	¼ cup
Granulated fructose	2 tablespoons
Raisins	½ cup
Whole-Grain cereal	2 ½ cups Wheaties®, Total®, or any other whole-grain, flaky cereal

Blend the first three ingredients in a small bowl. Separately, stir the next five ingredients together in a medium-size bowl. Add the blended dry ingredients, and mix together just until moist (not smooth). Add the raisins and cereal and fold together until the cereal is moistened. Make twelve regular-size muffins, filling each muffin cup about level with the top of the pan. (If any cups remain unfilled, put ¼ inch of cool tap water in those cups so the muffins cook evenly.) Bake in a preheated oven at 400° for about 20 minutes, until the muffins brown a little on top and spring back completely when touched with a finger or spoon.

Swheaties Muffins

If you prefer a sweeter muffin, double the granulated fructose to $1/4$ cup.

Oatbran Muffins

The list of ingredients below includes no oat bran. This is not a mistake. Rolled oats are 40% oat bran. Oats lack the gluten that makes bread rise and that holds the bubbles formed from the leavening agent; so these muffins are dense. They make good traveling companions, because they pack so much nourishment in a small space.

Ingredient	Amount
Quick-cooking rolled oats	$2\,1/4$ cups
or Hodgson Mills oat bran flour	$2\,1/4$ cups
Baking powder	2 teaspoons
NuSalt or salt	$1/2$ teaspoon

Preheat oven to 425°. Mix ingredients well in large bowl. Add:

Chopped walnuts	$1/4$ cup
Raisins	$1/4$ cup
Honey	$1/3$ cup
Skim milk, Lactaid milk, or nonfat plain yogurt	$1/2$ cup
Canola oil	2 tablespoons

Mix just until moistened. Fill a dozen muffin cups full. Bake 15 to 20 minutes or until just turning golden brown on top.

Texas-Size Cranberry-Orange Muffins

Spray the muffin pan with a cooking spray (oil) that you like or drop a quarter teaspoon of canola oil into each muffin cup and smear it around with your finger. (Or use ordinary smallish waxed-paper muffin liners and expect that you'll have to do a little scooping with a knife.) Preheat the oven to 375°.

I. Ingredient	Amount
Fresh or frozen cranberries	1 cup
Granulated fructose	2 tablespoons
Freshly grated orange peel	2 teaspoons

If using fresh cranberries, wash them and pick out any dark or bruised ones. Mix the good berries with the fructose in a saucepan (metal or range-safe ceramic), heat to boiling, and boil a minute or two until the cranberries have popped. For microwaving, put the ingredients in a quart glass or ceramic bowl, cover well, and microwave on High for 5 minutes or until the cranberries have popped and are soft. Let cool for 5 minutes. Add the orange peel and set aside.

If using frozen, chopped cranberries, mix the three ingredients in a bowl and set aside.

II. Ingredient	Amount
Flour	2 cups
Granulated fructose	¼ cup
Baking powder	2 teaspoons
NuSalt or salt	½ teaspoon

Blend these dry ingredients with a fork till well mixed.

III. Ingredient	Amount
Canola oil	2 tablespoons
Orange juice	½ cup
Egg substitute	½ cup (equals two eggs)
Wheat berries or wheat germ	¼ cup

In a small bowl, mix these ingredients together. Then pour them onto the dry ingredients and stir just until moistened, 25 strokes at most. Add the cranberry-orange mix and fold it in for a few strokes. Divide the batter evenly into the six muffin cups. Bake 25 to 30 minutes or until the tops brown slightly and rebound well when poked lightly with a wooden spoon. Let the muffins cool for 5 minutes in the pan before turning them out. Serve warm.

―――――――――――

Pineapple-Oatmeal Quickbread

I. Ingredient	Amount
Oatmeal	1 cup
Sour skim milk or buttermilk	1 cup

Heat and mix till thick and smooth. Cool to lukewarm.

II. Ingredient	Amount
Egg substitute	1/4 cup
Molasses	1 teaspoon
Granulated fructose	1/4 cup
Lemon extract	1/4 teaspoon
Canned crushed pineapple	two 8-ounce cans

Blend these wet ingredients together with the oat-dairy mix.

III. Ingredient	Amount
White flour	2 cups
NuSalt	1/2 teaspoon
Baking powder	1 tablespoon

Blend these dry ingredients together, then blend with the wet ingredients above just until moistened. Bake in a 9 x 5 x 3-inch pan at 375° or about 55 minutes, until the loaf browns a little on top and springs back completely when touched with a finger or spoon.

Pecan Rolls, Pecan-Raisin Rolls, and Cherry-Pecan Rolls

Ingredient	Amount
Dry yeast	1/2 package
Bread flour	1 1/8 cups
Hodgson's oat bran flour	1/2 cup
Honey	1/2 tablespoon
Walnut oil	1/2 tablespoon
Warm water	4 1/2 ounces
Salt or NuSalt	1/2 teaspoon
(Optional: Raisins or dried cherries 1/2 cup)	
Pecans, chopped	1/2 cup
Powdered sugar	1/2 cup
Ground cinnamon	1 1/2 teaspoons
Ground allspice	1/2 teaspoon

Knead and cycle the first seven ingredients through a breadmaker as for white bread. The oat bran absorbs water slowly, so at first the dough should look wet and sticky. Poke a finger into the dough lightly when there's about 10 more minutes of the last kneading left. If it seems tough and doesn't stick to your finger at all, add a tablespoon of water, let it mix a minute, and retest. If it's very sticky, add a tablespoon of flour, let it mix for a minute, and retest.

As soon as the second kneading ends, pull the dough out of the mixer. If it is too sticky to handle easily, add a teaspoon of bread flour here and there so you can grab it. Sprinkle flour onto the surface on which it will be rolled. Spread the dough with a rolling pin to at least 9 x 12 inches on a flat surface. (A cool marble surface helps prevent sticking.) Cover with the sugar and spice mix. Spread the chopped nuts and raisins on top. Roll up carefully, pressing to eliminate air pockets. Cut the long, thin loaf in half. Cut each half into three equal lengths. Lightly grease a Texas-size muffin pan with walnut oil. Fill the muffin pan with cut lengths of rolled dough. Rub a few drops of walnut oil onto the top, cut surface of each. Cover with a wet plastic or wax paper sheet. Cover that with a dish towel. Let rise for an hour in an oven preheated to 150°, then turned off before the rolls are put in it. Bake in a preheated oven at 375° for 25 minutes.

Turn rolls out of pan while still hot so the sugar doesn't make them stick to the pan. Spread with buttercream icing (see Chapter 22). Makes six rolls.

Suggestion: Double the bread recipe (the first seven ingredients), separate the dough into halves when the second kneading ends, and use half for the rolls. Put the rest back into the breadmaker and use it to make a 1-pound loaf of oatmeal bread.

Whole-Grain Pancakes and Ovencakes

Ingredient	Amount to Serve Two
Your favorite whole-grain pancake mix (e.g., Hodgson Mill Buckwheat Pancake Mix)	³⁄₄ cup
Quick-cooking oats	¹⁄₄ cup
1% milk or soy milk	¹⁄₂ cup
Egg substitute	2 ounces (equivalent to 1 egg)
Canola oil	2 teaspoons
Raisins or other dry fruit	¹⁄₄ cup
Buttery-flavor cooking spray	

Implements

A bowl that holds at least one quart for two people, two quarts for four people, etc.

A tablespoon or soup spoon for mixing and for cleaning out the bowl.

A glass or ceramic baking pan, about 9" x 12".

PREPARATION FOR OVENCAKES. Preheat an oven or toaster-oven to 400°. Spray cooking spray into the baking pan for 5 seconds or until you can see a bubbly layer on the entire bottom surface. Shake a tablespoon of pancake mix onto it, and shake it around till all the cooking spray is covered well. Shake out the excess dry pancake mix and discard.

MIXING INGREDIENTS. For pancakes or ovencakes, mix milk, egg substitute, and oil with a spoon until homogenized. Add pancake mix and oats and mix just until well moistened. Fold in the dry fruit of your choice. Let stand a minute until the mixture thickens. It should become as thick as a milkshake, not stay thin like ordinary pancake mix. If it's not thick, add another 2 tablespoons of pancake mix and fold it in gently. Don't overmix and lose the bubbles that are forming.

BAKING THE OVENCAKE. If you want the simplicity of the oven recipe, when the mix is thick, gently pour it into the pretreated glass or ceramic pan. Even out the depth of the mix in the pan by tipping a little and shaking a little. The mix should be about $1/4$" to $3/8$" thick. Bake 8 minutes. Turn on the broiler element. Broil 3 to 5 minutes, until browning slightly on top. Remove from oven. With a sharp knife, cut the cake into eighths and free the edges from the sides of the pan. Use a spatula of about the same width as the slices of cake to remove one slice at a time.

GRILLING PANCAKES. Pancakes need a medium-high heat to brown properly. When a dry pan is preheated enough on the range, droplets of water flicked from your hand into the pan should dance in the pan. (Never flick water into hot oil! The spattering can burn you.) Add a teaspoon of canola or olive oil to the pan and spread it out by tipping the pan this way and that slightly.

Scoop up the pancake mix with a wooden or plastic spoon that holds a full ounce easily. Pour it out gently with a circulating motion so the thickness of the cake spreads evenly. Watch the cakes. They should start drying on the edges before the edges look or smell burned. Change the heat setting if neither one happens within 2 to 5 minutes. When the edges are all dried but the center is not, flip the cakes over, once, to brown the other side. Expect the second side to brown much more quickly than the first.

Refresh the pan with another teaspoon of oil for each set of pan-cakes, or they will stick or not brown properly.

Hold the pancakes, until serving, on an oven-safe dish in an oven at its lowest warming setting (about 150°). Avoid covering them or they will become soggy.

SERVING CAKES. Serve with a few bases and toppings. Bases: bread-spread, fat-free cream cheese, yogurt, sour cream, or ricotta. Toppings: your favorite syrups, all-fruit jams, or apple butter.

Hash Browns and Cranberries

Make cranberry sauce from 8 ounces of fresh cranberries, 4 ounces of fructose, and water to barely cover. Boil in a saucepan till most berries pop. Cool in the fridge till gooey and thick.

In advance, bake a medium to large Idaho potato. This takes about 45 minutes in a 450° oven; in a microwave, it takes 4 to 5 minutes on High, turning the potato over in the middle of the cooking period. Don't go completely by time: Thump the potato lightly after it stops sizzling, and stop microwaving for good only when the potato indents easily. If you have time to wait, let the potato cool. Once baked, potatoes can sit out overnight without deteriorating or spoiling. If you can't wait, cut the hot potato in half the long way, wait a minute, and don a protective mitt to handle it. Either way, the next step is to put a tablespoon of oil into a 10-inch skillet, heat the skillet on medium-high just until the oil gets hot, and sprinkle 3 to 6 shakes of Vegit®* into the oil. Take the potato and grate it directly into the pan. Spread the potato out to cover the skillet. Do it lightly: Don't squash the potato together! Turn the potato bits over as soon as you see some browning. Depending on how dry your potato is, browning can start in as little as a minute, so watch carefully. Sprinkle 1/4 teaspoon of sweet (not hot) Hungarian paprika onto the potato mix. Flip again when the other side starts to brown, and mix a bit to coat the potato well with the paprika. Yeah, it looks great; but the main thing is that it is now tasty in a way that won't attack your stomach.

Serving: Put 1/4 cup of cranberry sauce on one side of your plate, and put a 2-tablespoon scoop of nonfat sour cream in the middle of it. Add the hash browns to the plate last. Put a 1-tablespoon scoop of bread-spread in the middle of the hash browns.

*Caution: Vegit® contains some stomach offenders.

Cheese Biscuits

Ingredient	Amount	
	Two	**Four**
Bisquick®	½ cup	1 cup
Self-rising flour	½ cup	1 cup
Skim milk	⅜ cup	¾ cup
Lite sharp cheddar cheese, grated	½ cup	1 cup

This is an illustration of how to dilute out the saturated fat in Bisquick® and make ordinary high-fat, low-protein biscuits into a more nutritious dish.

Measure all ingredients into a small bowl. Mix with a fork, just until the large lumps disappear. The batter should be a little lumpy. With a soup spoon, drop rounded spoonfuls of the batter onto a nonstick cookie sheet. Bake in a preheated oven at 400° for 15 minutes, or at 450° for 10 minutes if you are in a hurry, or until the biscuits start to brown here and there.

Serve hot with breadspread to bolster the protein content further. Pile on a low-sugar or fruit-only jam, or eat with berries or other fruit, to complete a balanced breakfast.

Tofu Scramble

Per Serving

2 ounces extra-firm tofu

½ teaspoon olive or canola oil

2–3 ounces sliced fresh mushrooms (or a medium potato, precooked and chopped)

1 slice soy cheese

To taste: Bragg Liquid Aminos, soy sauce, or tamari

Chop the tofu into slices ¼-inch thick. Brown slightly in an oiled hot skillet. Add mushrooms and liquid flavoring (Bragg's, soy sauce, or tamari). Cover. Stir occasionally until the mushrooms change color and begin to soften, about 2 minutes. Add the slice of cheese on top. Reduce heat to simmer. Cover the skillet again and let stand for a minute for the cheese to soften. Before serving, season lightly with Hungarian paprika and white pepper as desired for color and tang.

Eat this high-protein dish with whole-grain toast and a low-acid fruit juice such as grape, apple, or pear juice.

Tofu Breakfast Sausage

Ingredient	Amount
Extra-firm tofu, drained	10.5-ounce package
Egg substitute	2 ounces (equivalent to 1 egg)
Wheat germ (toasted, sweetened)	$1/4$ cup
Whole wheat bread or cracker crumbs	$1/4$ cup
Sunflower seeds, finely ground	2 tablespoons
Dried sage	$1/2$ teaspoon
Dried thyme	$1/2$ teaspoon
Oregano	$1/2$ teaspoon
(Optional: fennel seed $1/4$ teaspoon)	
Vegit® *	$1/4$ teaspoon
NuSalt or salt	$1/2$–1 teaspoon
Freshly ground pepper	$1/2$ teaspoon

PREPARATION

Mash the tofu well. Mix all the ingredients together in a bowl, kneading by hand.

For sausage patties: Press the mix into patties the size of a thin hamburger.

For link sausages: If you have a pasta maker, remove the center of the tube pasta attachment. Put the kneaded mix in the machine. Extrude tofu links, cutting them at 2-inch lengths. If you don't have a pasta maker that makes tubes, cut a half-inch corner off the end of a tough plastic bag (a zip-locking bag is tough enough), put the kneaded mix inside, and squash it out into a cylinder on a cookie pan. Cut the mix into 2-inch links.

COOKING AND STORAGE

Place sausage in a steamer. Steam for 15 minutes. Remove from steamer 5 minutes after it has stopped steaming. If you must hurry and remove the links sooner, do so very carefully, with mitts on, so you don't get burned from the steam.

Makes a dozen links or four to six patties. They can be frozen and reheated. Whether fresh-steamed or frozen, before serving, brown the sausage to bring out the taste. Spray a small skillet with cooking spray or add a teaspoon of canola oil. Grill the links until browned.

*Caution: Vegit® contains some stomach offenders.

Tempeh Tots

Per Serving

1 ounce tempeh, cut into hunks about $\frac{1}{2}$-inch square by
   $\frac{1}{4}$- or $\frac{1}{3}$-inch thick

1 teaspoon olive oil

To taste: sesame seeds, Hungarian paprika, and salt or
   Bragg Liquid Aminos

In a hot, dry skillet, pour the olive oil, then the tempeh. Add sesame seeds, paprika, and Bragg's or salt to coat the tempeh. Cook until it starts browning. Flip to brown the other side. Serve with hash browns, whole-grain toast, or breakfast cakes and with a side dish of fruit.

Chapter 15

Ⱳhat's for Lunch?

Ᏺn the chapters to follow you'll find a good many recipes for soups and salads, and for each of the starch-based dishes—pasta, potatoes, and rice. Grab ideas from any or all chapters for good lunches.

In this chapter, I'll give you some general suggestions about how to break your fast again after you breakfast. The idea is to refresh and enjoy—not to bloat, fatten yourself, or make yourself sleepy.

Ⱨow Many Midday Meals Do You Need?

Maybe you follow the convention that lunch is at noon, and that's that. If that works for you—if you don't feel ravenous or groggy by 10 or 11 A.M.—fine.

On the other hand, if you eat a modest portion of one of my low-cal breakfasts and have a long, active morning, you may be pretty ticked off at me, because you feel pretty ticked off at everybody by late morning. When you start feeling hungry, do yourself a favor—have a snack. Make it one of those recommended in the High-Protein Snacks section in Chapter 12. Fruit is especially good, because it's handy.

What if you get hungry again in the afternoon? Let's say you've had a good lunch, and you still get hunger pains by 3 P.M. Don't blame your willpower or this book. Have another good snack. Just watch two things: Watch your portions, and watch how conveniently you keep snacks at your desk.

A handful of crackers or pretzels, maybe just half an ounce, will do wonders for your stomach for an hour or more. Don't leave a big supply of a crunchy snack food open on your desk as you work. The entire contents of the bag, or at least a few ounces of it, will somehow disappear in an hour. Then you will find that, no matter how low-fat the snack is, it puts fat on you over a period of months. Instead, take out a handful of your snack, put it down, reseal the snack-food bag, and put it out of sight.

ℋOW PASTA PASTES YOU

It's hard not to be set up for afternoon sleepiness. From 1 to 3 P.M., we are at our sleepiest of the entire day except for bedtime. Making this worse, the latest research shows that most Americans undersleep by one or two hours a night. That really sets you up for needing a siesta.

How do you know if you are undersleeping? Our bodies usually remind us of this in three ways. We waken slowly in the morning, only with a struggle or with caffeine; we feel sleepy in the afternoon; and we tend to fall asleep when we are relaxing in the evening. One easy way to tell is this: If you must rely on an alarm clock or another person to wake you up in the morning, you are undersleeping.

Is undersleeping bad for us? Probably, yes, but it mainly affects our moods. Sleep deprivation causes irritability. German researchers found that one's cuss-count rises dramatically after undersleeping. If you react to small upsets more quickly and more hotly than you'd like, try sleeping more each night.

Now, let's get back to lunch. The problem with a high-carbohydrate lunch is that it makes more serotonin form in your brain.

What do pasta or potatoes have to do with a transmitter in your brain that is derived from an amino acid? It's complicated and it's indirect, but there is an effect. It's good for relieving anxiety or depression, but it also makes you sleepy. It's okay to have pasta as part of your lunch, but do put a good supply of protein in there too—some meat, cottage cheese, yogurt, beans, or tofu. You need a substantial supply of protein to prevent you from feeling mentally fuzzy or from falling asleep at your desk or from having too slow a reaction time when you're behind the wheel of your car.

Sandwiches

If you think that, after all this nutritional mumbo-jumbo, I'm going to tell you that you ought to have something as simple, as utterly ordinary, as a *sandwich* for lunch. . . well, I am.

Made right, a sandwich can be an ideal lunch. Put some high-protein foods in the middle, as I've suggested. Or go exotic and use tabbouli (See Chapter 16, Salad Specials) or baba ganoush. Salad ingredients are especially good for adding juiciness, flavor, and complete nutrition. Put the sandwich on whole-grain bread for more nutrition and slower digestion.

Skip the condiments, especially the spicy ones like mustard and the fatty ones like regular mayo, to help your stomach and your heart. If your sandwich is too dry for you, cover one or both slices of the bread with breadspread or plain yogurt or fat-free mayonnaise, or sprinkle a little salad vinegar on the salad greens in your sandwich.

If you like a "salad" sandwich—I mean, chicken salad or tuna salad—you can make some delicious versions without mayo. Start with finely chopped white-meat chicken or tuna packed in water.

For tuna, open the can, letting the lid fall into the can. Squeeze out the water by inverting the can and squeezing the lid onto the tuna. Remove the lid with a knife—don't break your nails. Add some tap water, mix a little, and squeeze again if you want to cut the fishiness of the taste and remove more salt.

Put 3 ounces of fat-free cream cheese in a small (cereal) bowl. Add 2 tablespoons of skim milk. Mix with a fork. Or use 4 ounces of plain yogurt if you like a more tart mix. Add 3 ounces of the chicken or tuna.

If you want to make the salad more exotic, add a dash of ground salad herbs, rosemary, or tarragon. Dress up your sandwich with salad greens, tomato slices, or whatever you like from the plant kingdom.

Don't succumb to the temptation of the peanut-butter-and-jelly alternative. That particular combo is comforting, but it's extremely high in fat and high in sugar.

What about reduced-fat peanut butter? Sorry, but after tasting the stuff, I can't recommend it. Besides, it still has three-quarters of the fat of regular peanut butter. I even tried a brand with "78 percent less fat than peanut butter." It had at least 78 percent less flavor than peanut butter, and it sits in my refrigerator still, untouched and unloved.

Soy butter works, but it's strong-tasting. Spread it thinner than the jelly (Polaner's or other fruit spread) on a soy-butter-and-jelly sandwich.

$\mathcal{W}$HAT YOU GET FROM SOUPS AND SALADS

Soups and salads provide many a good nutrient, especially vitamins and minerals. They can have surprisingly high protein levels too. They fill you up nicely because of their large volume. Finally, the warmth of soup and the chewiness of a salad each provide a special kind of eating satisfaction.

Don't expect them to get you through a long, busy afternoon, however. Except for heavy cream soups, soup is quite low-cal, about 100 calories in a good-size bowl. (Heavy cream soups have more calories, but of course they're not featured in this book because of their high fat content.) So pretend you're in a soup kitchen: Supplement it with bread. Make it whole-grain bread.

$\mathcal{S}$OUPS

The French call soup a "restaurant" (with the accents on the first and last syllables) because it is so nutritious that it is restorative. The name stuck to the establishments that served these bowls of liquid food. Nowadays, you can go to a restaurant that serves no restaurant. How strange.

As I emphasized earlier, there is one thing about most modern-day soups that is unhealthful—the huge amounts of salt they usually contain. In this era of epidemic stress and epidemic hypertension, it is important to make soup that is flavorful on its own without resorting to 8 or 10 grams of salt per serving.

The soups described below are each distinctive but not, I hope, weird. Eating them with crusty bread is important to make them truly restorative. There are not many calories in most vegetables.

Split-Pea Vegetable Soup

This soup is homage to my mom's split-pea soup, my childhood favorite. Except for substituting turkey Canadian bacon for a ham bone, to cut the fat and salt, and for adding the pickling spice, this is her soup.

About the pickling spice: If you object to little round seeds in your soup, be sure to mash or grind them up with a mortar and pestle or pepper grinder before adding them to the soup. They do soften on cooking, though.

Ingredient	Amount
Russet potato	1 medium
Whole baby carrots	4 ounces
Stalk celery	one
Green split peas	6 ounces, dry
Onion	1/4 cup, chopped and presoaked in water for 10 minutes
Pickling spice	1/4 teaspoon, ground
Turkey Canadian bacon, sliced	1/4 pound
Hot water	one quart
(If you have leftover stock from a New England Boiled Dinner, use that and cut the amount of plain water to make a total of one quart of liquid)	
Sweet fruit juice (grape, apple, etc.)	1 tablespoon
Salt	1 teaspoon or to taste

Put the water into a 3- to 5-quart pot or casserole. Peel the potato and slice it about 1/2 to 3/4 inch thick. A medium potato makes four to six slices. Immediately put the potato slices into the water so they don't turn brown. Chop the celery into bite-size pieces. Drain the chopped, pre-soaked onion. Chop the Canadian bacon into little bits or shreds. Add all ingredients to the pot except the salt, which is reserved until after the salt cooks out of the Canadian bacon. Heat the mix to boiling, and simmer for an hour. Keeping the pot on simmer, use a wire whisk, a wire pastry crust mixer, or a big fork to mash the potato and the carrots a little, without removing them from the pot. The peas should dissolve easily, not elude your smashing tool. If they still look like peas, keep simmering until they dissolve easily. The idea is to give the soup body and bits of color, not to homogenize the soup. Now drip a little of the soup onto a cold soupspoon and taste it. If it tastes flat, add a quarter teaspoon of salt and retest till satisfied. If it tastes bitter, add a tablespoon of the fruit juice, and retest.

Seafood Chowder Manhattan

This soup is quite hearty, even without the optional shrimp. Add crusty bread on the side, and it's a full meal. If tomatoes bother you, add the milk to neutralize the acid.

Ingredient	Amount
Fish fillets	1 pound
Turkey Canadian bacon, thin-sliced	1 ounce
Onion (Vidalia, Texas Sweet, green, green, or knob)	1/4 cup
Carrots, thin-sliced	2 medium
Dried parsley flakes	1 tablespoon
Fresh tomatoes, chopped	1 large or 2 small
Bay leaf	1 leaf
Crushed thyme	1 1/2 teaspoons
Medium potatoes, cubed	3
White wine	1 1/2 ounces
Optional: Deveined shrimp, 1/2 pound; skim milk, 1/4 to 1/2 cup	

Chop onion finely and soak in 1 cup hot water for at least 10 minutes. In a small skillet, brown the turkey Canadian bacon with 1 teaspoon of canola oil until crisped. Let cool slightly. Chop. Drain the water off the onions. Put 2 quarts of water in a soup pot; heat at medium. Add all the ingredients, Bring to a boil, reduce heat, and simmer 10 minutes or until the potato pieces and the fish fillets break easily with a fork. Taste carefully. Correct the seasoning with 1 to 1 1/2 teaspoons of salt or NuSalt and 1/8 to 1/4 teaspoon of pepper. If the soup is too strong or if desired for creaminess, add 1/4 to 1/2 cup of nonfat milk.

Tasty Lentil Soup

This soup is just plain distinctive. It doesn't taste like an imitation of anything else. You may find it calls for crackers as an accompaniment rather than bread such as SnackWells pepper crackers and breadspread.

Ingredient	Amount
Lentils	1 cup
Water	4 cups

In a soup pot, boil the lentils for 20 minutes without salt. Add:

Parsley Patch® seasoning*	1–2 teaspoons*
Carrots, diced	1 large or 2 small
Potato, diced	1 medium
Tomatoes, chopped	1 pound

Heat until the soup returns to a boil. Simmer 15–20 minutes. Add:

Chopped fresh mushrooms	4 ounces

Cook another 2–3 minutes.

Season to taste with 1–2 teaspoons of salt or NuSalt, $1/8$–$1/4$ teaspoons of pepper, 1 teaspoon of coriander, and $1/2$–2 teaspoons of Bragg Liquid Aminos or soy sauce. Avoid adding too much soy; it overpowers the other tastes.

*Caution: Add Parsley Patch® seasoning with care, or delete it from the recipe if some contents might offend your stomach. It is a blend of spices, baker's yeast, whey, onion, chili pepper, tomato, garlic, red pepper, lemon peel, and jalapeno.

Greens and Beans Soup

Please don't be put off by the weird-looking addition of Lapsang Souchong tea to this soup. The tea adds a hint of smoky sweetness, but nothing objectionable.

Ingredient	Amount
Dried white beans	$1/2$ pound
Olive oil	$1/2$ tablespoon
Chopped onion	$1/4$ cup
Bay leaf 1 leaf	
Fresh dark greens—escarole, kale, or spinach	3 ounces, chopped
Carrots	$1/2$ cup
Lapsang Souchong tea	2 bags

Soak beans overnight at room temperature in 2 quarts of cold water. Presoak the chopped onion in hot water for at least 10 minutes. Drain. In a soup pot, heat the olive oil and onions on medium. Cook until lightly browned. Drain beans. Add beans and 1 $\frac{1}{2}$ quarts hot water to the soup pot. Add bay leaf. Heat to boiling. Reduce heat. Simmer, partially covered, until beans are tender, 1 $\frac{1}{2}$ to 2 hours. Add hot water as needed to keep the soup from congealing.

Add carrots and tea bags. Simmer 15 minutes. Remove tea bags. Add salt or NuSalt, pepper, and greens. Simmer 1 to 3 minutes until greens turn dark and barely become tender. Correct the seasoning.

To serve, sprinkle with grated parmesan cheese.

Potato-Cheese Soup

This soup is fast, easy, nutritious, filling, and very comforting to a stomach that has been upset recently. Try it on a cold evening after you've been under serious stress all day at work.

Ingredient	Amount
Canola oil	1 teaspoon
Vegit®*	$\frac{1}{8}$ teaspoon
Water	$\frac{1}{2}$ cup
Idaho potato	1 medium or large
Carrot	1 small
Nonfat milk and hot water	1 cup each
Grated nonfat or low-fat cheddar cheese	$\frac{1}{2}$ cup
White pepper	$\frac{1}{8}$–$\frac{1}{4}$ teaspoon, to taste
Salt or NuSalt	$\frac{1}{4}$–$\frac{1}{2}$ teaspoon, to taste

Put the oil in a 10-inch skillet. Sprinkle 3 to 6 shakes of Vegit into the oil. Heat for half a minute. Grate the carrot into the skillet. Add $\frac{1}{2}$ cup water and simmer for 3 to 5 minutes, until carrot is tender. Bake a medium or large Idaho potato about 45 minutes at 450° in an oven or 4 to 5 minutes in the microwave on High, turning the potato over in the middle of the cooking period. Quit baking or microwaving only when the potato indents easily. If you have time to wait, let it cool. If you can't wait, cut the hot potato in half the long way, wait a minute, and don a protective mitt to handle it. Grate the potato directly into the skillet. Add the cup of nonfat milk and the cup of water. Heat to boiling. Add the grated cheese last and don't reboil; just stir until the cheese melts in (otherwise, it forms a grainy glop). Season with pepper and salt. Serve immediately. To garnish, sprinkle with dried parsley. Serve with oyster crackers or bread sticks.

*Caution: Vegit® contains some stomach offenders.

New-Fashioned Chicken-Rice Soup

This chicken soup is just as nutritious as the old-fashioned kind, but it has less fat and less salt. It combines low-fat chicken, plenty of vegetables, rice, and several unexpected tastes to make a satisfying, tantalizing repast all by itself. Try making this one for a winter party and see how fast it disappears.

Ingredient	Amount
Canola oil	1 teaspoon
Whole Amish chicken, 3 1/2–4 pounds	1
Chopped sweet onion	1/2 cup
Chopped carrot	1 cup
Chopped celery stalks	2
Wild rice	3 ounces
Lundberg Wild Blend Rice	6 ounces
Celery seed	pinch
Clove	1 whole
Salt	2 teaspoons
Mixed peppercorns	10
Nutmeg	pinch
Tarragon	1/2 teaspoon
Low-salt beef bouillon crytstals	1 tablespoon
Sweet Hungarian paprika	1/2 teaspoon
Honey	1 teaspoon

Select Vidalia, walla walla, Texas Sweet, or green onions. Chop finely. Presoak in a cup of hot water for at least 10 minutes. Drain well. Put the teaspoon of canola oil into a soup pot that holds at least 10 quarts. Heat to medium-high. Brown the chicken, breast down, covered loosely, turning heat down to medium. When the chicken breast is well-browned, flip the chicken onto its back. Add the drained onion. Brown both the onion and the back of the chicken. Add a gallon of hot water, the rice, all the vegetables, and all the herbs and spices. Simmer for an hour and a half or until the chicken begins to fall off the bones.

Remove the chicken. Debone the meat and cut it into bite-size pieces. Add it back to the pot, along with:

Fresh asparagus	1/2 pound, cut into 1/2-inch pieces
Fresh mushrooms—half shiitake, half buttom mushrooms	1/2 pound, cut into 1/4-inch slices

Reheat to boiling and simmer until the asparagus is tender but still dark green, about 3 minutes. Serve with a light fresh bread and breadspread.

Chapter 16

SALAD SPECIALS

SEAFOOD SALADS

Salade Nicoise Pacific Northwest Style

This takes more time and effort than most recipes in this book, but it makes a large salad that is elegant enough to serve as the main dish for an al fresco dinner party.

Ingredient	Amount to Serve 2 to 3
Pacific Salmon	1/2 pound steak
Potatoes: new, red, or Idaho	3/4 pound
Fresh green beans	1/2 pound
Fresh wax beans	1/2 pounds
Fresh tomato	1 pound
Black olives	1/4 cup
Red leaf or romaine lettuce	1/2 head

Cover salmon with 1/2 teaspoon of dried, crushed tarragon. Coat salmon with 1 tablespoon breadspread or plain yogurt. Broil salmon for 15 minutes or until it just begins to flake and is pink in the center. Remove from broiler, remove skin and bones, and cut the salmon into bite-size pieces (or into long slices if you prefer). Cut potatoes into bite-size pieces. Boil for about 10 minutes, until a fork breaks them. (To microwave with water, see Boiled Red Potatoes in Chapter 19.) Remove from boiling water with a slotted spoon. Cool in a colander under running water. Set aside. Add the beans to the boiling water and boil till crisp-tender, about 7 minutes (or microwave with 1/4 cup water for 5 minutes on High and 2 minutes on Low). Cool the beans in the colander under running water.

Break half the leaves off a head of red lettuce. Wash the lettuce in cold water and shake dry (or spin dry in a salad spinner). Arrange leaves with the red ends out on a serving platter, a big shallow pasta bowl, or a big cutting board (anything larger than 9" x 12"). Arrange all the other ingredients on the lettuce. Put them in rows, in circles, or just in piles here and there.

Serve with smoked turkey dressing, tarragon vinaigrette, or dill dressing.

Lexa's Tuna Salad Casserole

Ingredient	Amount to Serve 2 to 3
Small shells pasta	4 ounces
Water	1 quart
Salt or NuSalt	1 teaspoon
Frozen baby peas	4 ounces
Canned tuna, water pack	6 ounces
Celery	1 stalk
Olive oil	1 tablespoon
Nonfat sour cream	4 ounces
LifeTime nonfat cheddar	2 ounces
Lemon	juice of 1 medium

Bring the salted water to a boil. Add the shells. Boil 8 minutes on medium, stirring occasionally so they don't stick together. Add the peas and boil for half a minute more. Pour into a colander and rinse once with cold water. Set aside.

While the shells are cooking, open the can of tuna and rinse the tuna lightly with tap water to get rid of the salty packing water. Put the tuna into a shallow bowl. With a fork, break the tuna into small chunks. Chop the celery and the cheddar into quarter-inch cubes.

In a 2-quart casserole, toss the shells, peas, celery, tuna, and cheese with the oil, sour cream, and lemon juice. Chill. Serve on lettuce with a salad dressing of your choice.

VEGETARIAN SALADS

To make a main dish out of a salad, it needs a source of carbohydrate. Pasta salads are popular, of course. Their fat content can be exorbitant, though. Potato salads can give more variety than you might guess.

Whole wheat berries (bulgur wheat) cooked slightly and flavored with herbs make tabouli, a fine complement to salad greens. Its nutty taste can easily get lost in Middle Eastern recipes, which tend to smother it in onions, cucumbers, and garlic. Try the following tabouli recipes for a satisfying lunch salad, or as a filling for sandwiches.

Tabouli #1—Very Veggie

This is not even remotely authentic, but it's wonderful for you and tastes very pleasant. It is much more tolerable for sensitive stomachs than authentic tabouli. It uses substitutes for chick peas, cucumbers, garlic, mint, and spices, and it tones down the onion. It substitutes a delicious surprise for lemon juice. The parsley comforts the stomach.

Ingredient	Amount to Serve 6
Bulgur wheat	3/4 cup (4 1/2 ounces)
Hot water	2 cups
Fresh tomatoes	1/2 pound
Fresh parsley	1 bunch (2 cups chopped)
Onion: Vidalia, Texas Sweet, or green	1/4 cup, chopped
Optional:Vegit®*	1 teaspoon
Frozen baby peas	1 cup
Salt or NuSalt	1 teaspoon
Black pepper, ground	1/4 teaspoon
Lemon juice, freshly squeezed, or apple cider vinegar	(See instructions.)

Prepare the onions first. Use Vidalia or Texas Sweet onion unless you don't tolerate them. If you don't, but you tolerate green onion, use that. Soak either for at least an hour in a full cup of cold water, preferably overnight. (Soak 5 to 10 minutes in hot water if you are in a hurry.) Pour off all the water before adding the onion to the recipe. If you don't tolerate any raw onion, use Vegit® * to taste. About 1 teaspoon will be needed to give enough flavor.

Put the bulgur in a 2-quart casserole. Add the 2 cups of hot water. Let stand 30 minutes or until soft. A faster way is to heat to near boiling; then let stand 10 minutes. As it stands, chop the tomatoes and parsley.

Drain bulgur well, but don't squeeze it. Drain onion. Put all ingredients in a large mixing bowl. Toss well. Refrigerate to store.

*Caution: Vegit® contains some stomach offenders.

About 5 or 10 minutes before serving the tabouli, make final preparations. Take a cup of tabouli per person and put it in a bowl. Add the apple cider vinegar or lemon juice, toss, and let it stand to absorb the juice. Use lemon juice if you want an unreserved tang and if your stomach tolerates lemon juice. Use apple cider vinegar if you want a mix of tang and sweetness or if you tolerate it better. An unpasteurized cider vinegar such as Hain is the tastiest, but plain old Heinz is fine too. Serve on romaine lettuce leaves with wedges of pita bread. If using in sandwiches, spread whole wheat, rye, or pumpernickel pitas or thin slices of bread, English muffins, or bagels with plain yogurt and heap on the tabouli.

Tabouli #2—Nuttier and More Filling

Ingredient	Amount to Serve 6
Bulgur wheat	¾ cup (4 ½ ounces)
Hot water	2 cups
Fresh tomatoes	¼ pound
Fresh parsley	½ bunch (1 cup chopped)
Onion: Vidalia, Texas Sweet, or green	¼ cup, chopped
Optional: Vegit®*	1 teaspoon
Pecans or walnuts, raw	¼ cup, chopped
Salt or NuSalt	½ teaspoon
Black pepper, ground	⅛ teaspoon
Lemon juice, freshly squeezed, or apple cider vinegar	(See instructions.)

Make and serve tabouli as above. When using this as a sandwich filling, spread the bread or pita with some plain yogurt first, and add lettuce.

*Caution: Vegit® contains some stomach offenders.

Couscous Tabouli

Couscous is Moroccan pasta, nothing more than bits of spaghetti. It is so small that it takes no more cooking time than bulgur does (see previous recipes). If you want a tabouli-like salad but don't want all that whole-wheat taste, make tabouli as in either recipe above but substitute cous-

cous for half or all of the bulgur. If you make it with half bulgur, it will have a stronger taste, of course. The all-couscous version can be made tastier, too. Just add 2 teaspoons of your favorite bouillon crystals—chicken, beef, or vegetarian—to the hot water before you use it to soften (cook) the couscous.

Sesame Noodles

Ingredient	Amount to Serve 4
Angel hair, spaghetti, or linguine	1/2 pound
Onion to flavor	(See tabouli recipes.)
Broccoli 1/2 head	(about 4 ounces)
Mushrooms	6 large, sliced (about 4 ounces)
Bragg Liquid Aminos and Sesame Oil	1 tablespoon each
Kikkoman Light Soy Sauce	1 teaspoon
Cilantro, fresh, chopped	1 tablespoon
Optional: Use fresh chopped parsley or basil, 1 tablespoon, if you don't like the taste of cilantro.)	
Sesame seeds, toasted	2 tablespoons

Prepare onion as in tabouli recipes. Boil noodles in about 2 quarts of water with a teaspoon each of olive oil and salt. Cook until the noodles are as soft as you like. Drain. Wash with cold tap water.

As the noodles cook, chop the broccoli into bite-size pieces. Steam just until it turns dark green, about 5 minutes. Add mushrooms. Steam for another 3 minutes or until the 'shrooms darken a little and the broccoli is crisp-tender. Wash in cold tap water.

Put the drained pasta, the mushrooms and broccoli, and the "onion to flavor" in a large serving bowl. Blend the Bragg's, the soy, and the sesame oil in a cup. Pour it on the pasta and vegetables. Add the cilantro and sesame seeds. Toss. Can be served immediately, but the flavor and texture improve on standing, covered and refrigerated, for an hour or overnight. Serve over fresh greens.

Italian Pasta Salad

Ingredient	Amount to Serve 4
Rigatone pasta	1/2 pound
Onion to flavor	(See tabouli recipes.)
Italian dressing (See Salad Dressings.)	1/4 cup
Chopped fresh tomato	1 small (about 4 ounces)
Mushrooms	6 large, sliced (about 4 ounces)
Olive oil	1 tablespoon
Fresh chopped basil leaves	1 tablespoon
Fresh chopped oregano leaves	1 tablespoon
Weight Watchers grated parmesan	1/4 cup

Prepare onions as in tabouli recipes. Boil noodles in about 2 quarts of water with a teaspoon each of olive oil and salt. Cook until the noodles are as soft as you like. Drain. Wash with cold tap water. As the noodles cook, wash and chop the tomato into bite-size pieces and slice the mushrooms. Put the drained pasta and the vegetables in a large serving bowl. Pour the Italian dressing and the olive oil on the pasta and vegetables. Add the basil, oregano, and parmesan. Toss. Can be served immediately, but the flavor and texture improve on standing, covered and refrigerated, for at least an hour or overnight.

Grilled Chicken Salad

Ingredient	Amount to Serve 4
Skinless chicken breast halves (Amish)	2
Sage, ground	1 teaspoon
Rosemary, ground	1 teaspoon
Hellman's fat-free mayonnaise	1–2 tablespoons, as needed to cover chicken
Salad greens	4 cups
Berry vinaigrette	(See Salad Dressings.)

Wash chicken carefully in running water. Cover breasts with sage and rosemary. With a table knife, spread the mayo over the seasonings and the chicken, taking care not to reach back into the mayo jar after it has touched the chicken. Grill in a toaster oven at 450° degrees just until no pink color shows in the middle. As the chicken broils, make a green salad big enough for four people. Let chicken cool until warm, not hot. Debone if it was bone-in. Chop into bite-size pieces. Spread the pieces over the salad. Serve with raspberry or blueberry vinaigrette dressing and with crusty bread or breadsticks and breadspread or olive oil.

Salad Dressings

Don't rely on Kraft or Mama Marzetti all the time—make your own salad dressings. It takes only a couple of minutes to create something not just good, but great. Do not be put off by your lack of expertise compared to the chef at some big company.

There isn't much to learn. Read a salad dressing label, and you'll find only five necessities. One is to give bite, maybe vinegar. Something sweet balances the sour. Something makes it stick to the salad vegetables (creams and oils both work). Something gives spicy tastes, especially pepper. And of course there is salt, the universal flavor enhancer. American salad dressings also usually include some onion and garlic.

With this in mind, make a salad and leave aside a few bits of lettuce or whatever is the mildest part of your salad. These are for sampling with your dressing as you correct its seasoning to your taste. Don't expect to get the flavor of the dressing just right on the very first try, before you correct the seasonings.

Now make your salad dressing. Let freshness be your secret weapon. Make a fresh dressing every time you serve a salad. Make plenty for one salad, but not enough to store and use again and again. Allow 2 ounces of dressing per person, less for a small side salad. Start by putting the creamy or watery part in a round-bottomed cup. Add the vinegar or other sour liquid. Mix with a fork. Crush the herbs. You can do so one herb at a time in the palm of your hand, kneading with your opposite thumb or the knuckle of your index finger; or you can crush them all together in a mortar with a pestle. You don't have to powder the herbs, just break them up a bit so they release more of their essence. Then add the herbs to the liquids and mix with a fork. That's all there is to it.

Honey-Mustard Yogurt Dressing

Ingredient	Number Served			
	One	**Two**	**Four**	**Your Way**
Honey	1/2 teaspoon	1 teaspoon	2 teaspoon	_____
Warm water	1 teaspoon	2 teaspoons	4 teaspoons	_____
Plain vinegar	1 tablespoon	2 tablespoons	4 tablespoons	_____
Dijon mustard	1/2 teaspoon	1 teaspoon	2 teaspoons	_____
Yogurt	1 tablespoon	2 tablespoons	4 tablespoons	_____
Salt or NuSalt	pinch	2 pinches	1/4 teaspoon	_____

In a cup, mix the honey with the water first, using a teaspoon. Then add the other ingredients and beat with a fork for 15 or 20 seconds. Dip a bit of lettuce into the dressing and taste it. If it's too salty, sour, or strong (mustardy), add another 2 tablespoons of yogurt. If it's too sweet, add another 1/2 teaspoon of vinegar. Try tasting some lettuce with the dressing again. Following these directions, keep correcting the dressing to your taste. Then cross out the amounts above and add your versions in the "Your Way" column.

Try this on a green salad with tiny shrimp tossed in.

Celery Seed Dressing

Ingredient	Number Served			
	One	**Two**	**Four**	**Your Way**
Fat-free sour cream	1 ounce	1/4 cup	1/2 cup	_____
Honey	1/2 teaspoon	1 teaspoon	2 teaspoons	_____
Olive oil	1 teaspoon	2 teaspoons	4 teaspoons	_____
Apple cider vinegar	1 tablespoon	2 tablespoons	1/4 cup	_____
White vinegar with tarragon	1 tablespoon	2 tablespoons	1/4 cup	_____
Celery seed	1/2 teaspoon	1 teaspoon	2 teaspoons	_____
Savory	1/4 teaspoon	1/2 teaspoon	1 teaspoon	_____
Tarragon	1/4 teaspoon	1/2 teaspoon	1 teaspoon	_____

	One	Two	Four	Your Way
Optional (contains stomach offenders): Pritikin or other fat-free Italian dressing	1 teaspoon	2 teaspoons	4 teaspoons	_____

Ranch Dressing

Leave out the celery seed, savory, and tarragon in the Celery Seed recipe. Substitute minced dill weed. If using dry dill weed, use $1/2$ teaspoon per person. If using fresh dill weed, use $1/8$ teaspoon per person.

Bacon Dressing

Ingredient	Amount to Serve 4
Turkey Canadian bacon, thin-sliced	$1/4$ pound
Canola oil	1 teaspoon

Make Ranch dressing, omitting the dill. Pour the oil into a 10-inch skillet. At medium heat, brown the Canadian bacon till crispy. Remove the bacon from the pan. Chop it finely with a large, sharp knife. Add to the ranch dressing. Use in place of bacon dressing on spinach salads.

Hot Bacon Dressing

Ingredient	Amount to Serve 4
Vidalia or Texas Sweet onion	2 thin slices
Turkey ham or Canadian bacon	2 ounces
Canola oil	1 teaspoon
Hot water	5 ounces
Honey	2 teaspoons

| Apple cider vinegar | 1 tablespoon |
| Chicken bouillon powder | 1/2 teaspoon |

In a 10-inch skillet, saute the ham or bacon and onion in the canola oil until they start to brown. Add 2 tablespoons of water, bring to a boil, and brown the onions till soft and tan. Add 1/2 cup of water, the bouillon powder, vinegar, and honey. Bring to a boil. Serve hot with a spinach or other salad, or pour over baked potatoes.

Blueberry or Raspberry Vinaigrette Dressing

Ingredient	Number Served			
	One	**Two**	**Four**	**Your Way**
Fresh or frozen blueberries or raspberries	9	18	36	_____
Cold water	1 tablespoon	2 tablespoons	1/4 cup	_____
Apple cider vinegar	1 tablespoon	2 tablespoons	1/4 cup	_____
Walnut (or canola) oil	1 teaspoon	2 teaspoons	1 tablespoon	
Salt or NuSalt	pinch	1/8 teaspoon	1/4 teaspoon	_____
Italian seasoning mix	1/4 teaspoon	1/2 teaspoon	1 teaspoon	_____
Vegit®*	1/4 teaspoon	1/2 teaspoon	1 teaspoon	_____
Honey	1/4 teaspoon	1/2 teaspoon	1 teaspoon	_____

In a cup, mash the berries with a fork. Add the water and mash again. Add the other ingredients. Beat with a fork for 15 or 20 seconds. Dip a bit of lettuce into the dressing and taste it. If it's too salty or sour, add 1/4 teaspoon of honey. If it's too sweet, add another tablespoon of vinegar. If it tastes too strong for you, add 2 tablespoons of water.

Berry-flavored vinaigrettes are especially good on green salads with chicken.

*Caution: Vegit® contains some stomach offenders.

Babe's Blue Cheese Dressing

Ingredient	Number Served			
	One	Two	Four	Your Way
Fat-free mayonnaise, Hellman's or Eden's	1 tablespoon	1 ounce	2 ounces	_____
Fat-free sour cream	1 tablespoon	1 ounce	1/4 cup	_____
Nonfat milk	1/2 tablespoon	1 tablespoon	2 tablespoons	_____
Dill weed	pinch	1/4 teaspoon	1/2 teaspoon	_____
White pepper, freshly ground	1/2 tablespoon	1 tablespoon	1 ounce	_____
Blue cheese, crumbled	1/2 tablespoon	1 tablespoon	1 ounce	_____

In a cup, beat all ingredients except blue cheese with a fork for half a minute or until smooth. Add the blue cheese and mix just enough to distribute the cheese evenly.

Blue cheese dressing is especially good on bitter greens.

Italian Dressing

Ingredient	Number Served		
	Two	Four	Your Way
Apple cider vinegar	2 tablespoons	1/4 cup	_____
Water	1 tablespoon	2 tablespoons	_____
Olive oil	2 teaspoons	4 teaspoons	_____
Hellman's fat-free mayonnaise	1 tablespoon	2 tablespoons	_____
Italian seasoning mix	1/4 teaspoon	1/2 teaspoon	_____
Vegit®*	1/4 teaspoon	1/2 teaspoon	_____
Salt or NuSalt	1/4 teaspoon	1/2 teaspoon	_____

In a cup, mix the ingredients and beat with a fork for 15 or 20 seconds. Dip a bit of lettuce into the dressing and taste it. If it's too tasteless, add another pinch of salt. If it's too salty or sour, add 1/4 teaspoon of sugar. If it's too strong, add another 2 tablespoons of water. Mix again. Try tasting some lettuce with the dressing again. Following these directions, keep correcting the dressing to your taste. Then cross out the amounts above and add your versions in the "Your Way" column.

Caution: Vegit® contains some stomach offenders.

Chapter 17

ℬREADS AND PIZZAS

𝒯his chapter is about yeast-raised breads. Muffins and loaves of quickbread, which are raised with baking powder, are covered in Chapter 14 (What's for Breakfast?).

ℐELECTING A LOAF OF BREAD

Whole-grain bread always gives better nutrition, including essential amino acids, vitamins, minerals, and fatty acids. It also gives more taste. Experiment with different kinds of bread to decide which ones you like. Some, like rye, are strong-tasting and demand strong-tasting fillings or toppings. Light-tasting fillings get lost inside a sandwich made with rye bread. Some whole-grain breads are light-tasting, such as oat bread, and are sweeter, making them good for breakfast as well as for sandwiches. Some labels don't tell you much, such as "whole wheat." All this means is that it contains *some* whole wheat flour. The loaf may be all whole-wheat flour or much less than half whole wheat. The rest will be white flour. So, read the ingredients list. The ingredient present in the largest amount must be given first, and so on.

Fresh-baked bread from your local bakery is much more likely to please you than the pre-sliced stuff in the plastic bags with the famous names. The bakery bread will be fresher. It should have no preservatives. The ingredients lists provide another interesting contrast: The bakery bread may have no fats or oils added. The famous-name bread in the plastic bag is likely to have partially hydrogenated fat added. That helps keep it soft and spongy as it sits on the grocer's shelf. It also contributes to atherosclerosis.

ℱLAT BREADS

Pita bread looks like a little pizza minus the toppings. Broken in half and opened gently, it provides a pocket that fills neatly with sandwich makings. It can also be topped to make a quick pizza. Because it is all crust and has so much surface area, it can dry out fast. I first enjoyed pita bread in a Greek restaurant. Then I was frustrated to find that the pitas available in the grocery store were tough and stale in comparison. There is a way to refresh them, though. Run the pita under running water just for a moment. Drain it, and blot it lightly. Pop it into the microwave for 15 seconds (20 for large pitas). It should come out hot, moist, and "fresh." If it's too moist, put it in a toaster oven for a minute.

Another enjoyable flat bread is focaccia. This is an Italian bread that not only looks like a pizza dough, it *is* one. Focaccias always used to come with a little cheese on top. {I found that helps not only for taste but also for ballast, keeping the bread from blowing up in the middle like a huge pita.} Now they're sold as pizza crusts and tend to have lots of herbs in them. If you're sensitive to onions and garlic, read the labels carefully.

There are two other kinds of flat breads that are commonly available to us, very flat breads. One, of course, is the soft flour tortilla. Please don't confuse its nutritional value with that of the grease-soaked flour tortilla that is cooked into a bowl shape and used for Mexican-influenced salads. Even the plain tortillas tend to have more oils in them than ordinary bread, though, so read the label before you make your choice.

The worst part of this is that the oils used in breads are partially hydrogenated. This means they have artificial *trans* double-bonds instead of the natural *cis* double-bonds in good oils. The companies that make breads and ship them long distances want them to last a long time on the grocery store shelves. Oils with cis double bonds do not stay fresh for a long time; they turn rancid. That is why the partial hydrogenation is done. It is being increasingly recognized in nutritional and pharmaceutical circles, however, that partially hydrogenated oils are not foods, they are food additives and have pharmaceutical properties. They raise LDL, or bad cholesterol, for instance.

The other very flat bread is Indian flat bread. Some of these breads, papadam, are chock-full of black pepper, or salt, or both. So be careful; don't just gobble when you are in an Indian restaurant.

♂OASTING

There are a couple of good reasons to toast bread. One is to give more chewing satisfaction. Another is to renew bread to more of the taste it had when it was fresh. A third is to add new taste through browning. The browning process, which is highly mysterious even to biochemists, definitely adds taste. It does burn up a little of the carbohydrate and protein, though.

Don't use a toaster oven to toast bread unless no toaster is available or your bread is too thickly cut to fit into a toaster. Toaster ovens do not radiate heat as intensely as toasters do. They substitute for this by heating bread with hot air instead. This makes your bread dry out in a toaster oven. A toaster won't do this. It browns the bread on the outside and leaves it moist inside.

What if your bread is already too dry? Maybe you aren't French enough to shop for fresh bread every day. You could toast it stale. You'd get melba toast—very thick melba toast; melba toast so crusty it could cut your gums.

Or you can try resuscitating your bread. Do not try warming it in a wet bag. This old idea works once in a while, but not more often than that in my experience.

Instead, try this method. {If you're left-handed, reverse the hands used in the following procedure.) Hold a slice of bread in your left hand. Put your right hand under lukewarm running tap water. Now pretend you are in the bathroom, shaking water off your hand before drying it. Shake the water droplets onto the bread, distributing the water as evenly as you can. Do this two or three times, till the surface is about half-covered with water. Toast on a medium-dark setting. As the water steams out, it steams into the bread too, refreshing it. When the outside gets hot enough, it will toast.

♏AKING BREAD

BREAD BY THE LOAF: USING A BREADMAKER

Breadmakers are wonderful. They save you energy and time. They give you easy access to any special bread that you might want. And they produce great results—sometimes.

It's the "sometimes" that I've worked on for a couple of years. Here's the way to change that to "always." First, get a breadmaker that allows you to sample what's going on in the early stages. This does not mean getting a $300 version of a machine. You can do fine with a low-cost one such as the one available by mail-order from DAK catalogs.

Then, recognize that flour is highly variable in how compacted it is, how much air it has in it, and, for whole-grain flour, how much water it has in it. So no recipe can be exactly right or consistently applied. Always start with a ratio by volume of three parts of flour to one part of water. If you want a big loaf, use 3 cups of flour to 1 cup of water. If you want a small loaf, try 2 cups of flour to 2/3 cup water. Your breadmaker may start with bigger or smaller amounts, but you can't vary the quantity too much or it won't come out right. Now, expect that the amounts added will not be the last. Be prepared to add more of either quickly. Add flour or water a tablespoon at a time, not more, and let it mix for a minute before you resample.

Five minutes after the first kneading cycle starts, a basic loaf of white or wheat bread should have a certain consistency. It should stick together well, not to the chamber in which it's mixing. If it's too wet to stick together well, add more flour till it does. It should stick to your finger, but only barely. It should not act tough, audibly slowing the mixer's motor. If it flakes, won't stick to your finger whatsoever, or slows the motor, add more water.

Grains added in pieces big enough to see easily, such as rolled oats or wheat berries, are more tricky. They absorb less water at first and more over the first half hour. So, you have to resample during the second kneading and prepare to add more water then, or let the dough be very sticky during the first kneading (very tricky indeed).

The breadmakers come with basic recipes and many an exotic recipe. Here are three bits of advice: Start with their basic recipes and, with the precautions above, use them faithfully till you have the hang of it. Then try the single-addition recipes if you like molasses or apricots or whatever. Avoid the recipes that have two or more flavors added, because this confusion of flavors can be very tiresome in a food as basic as bread.

Here are a couple of recipes for specialty breads to whet your appetite for trying the whole idea.

Whole Wheat Bread

Ingredient	Amount
Bread flour or all-purpose flour	2 ¼ cups
Fresh whole wheat flour	¾ cup
Dry yeast	1 package
Warm (not hot) water	9 ounces
Salt	1 teaspoon
Canola oil	1–2 tablespoons (more gives softer bread)
Brown sugar	2 tablespoons, packed

Knead and cycle through the breadmaker as for white bread. The dough should look wet and sticky at first. If it does, wait 10 minutes from the start to do anything about it. Then poke a wooden tool into the dough quickly and carefully. If it seems tough and doesn't stick to the tool at all, add a tablespoon of water, let it mix a minute, and retest. If it's sticky, add a tablespoon of flour, let it mix for a minute, and retest.

Bake to medium doneness. After it's baked, turn it out of the loaf pan immediately. If it's not browned well enough, heat an oven to 400°. Pop the loaf into the middle of the oven for 5 to 10 minutes, until the outside is evenly browned. After you remove the loaf from its last heating, do not cover it except loosely for the first 3 hours, so that the crust stays crispy.

The yeast removes most of the sugar that was added. This recipe makes about a 1 ½-pound loaf. The bread has about 0.7 gram fat per 1-ounce slice with 1 tablespoon of oil in the recipe.

Rye Bread

Substitute rye flour for the whole wheat flour; otherwise the recipe is the same.

Oatmeal-Maple Bread

Ingredient	Amount
Bread flour or all-purpose flour	2 ¼ cups
Hodgson Mill oat bran flour blend	¾ cup
Dry yeast	1 package

Warm (not hot) water	9 ounces
Salt	1 teaspoon
Canola oil	1 tablespoon
Dark maple syrup	2 tablespoons

Knead and cycle through breadmaker as for white bread. The oat bran absorbs water slowly, so at first the dough should look wet and sticky. If it does, wait till later to do anything about it. Poke a wooden tool into the dough when about 10 more minutes of the last kneading remain. If the dough seems tough and doesn't stick to your tool at all, add a tablespoon of water, let it mix a minute, and retest. If it's very sticky, add a tablespoon of flour, let it mix for a minute, and retest. Bake to medium doneness. After it's baked, do not cover it except loosely for the first 3 hours, so that the crust stays crispy.

This bread tastes interesting, but not sweet. The yeast removes most of the sugar from the maple syrup that is added. This recipe makes about a 1 ½-pound loaf. The bread has about 0.7 gram fat per 1-ounce slice.

Challah Bread

Ingredient	Amount
Bread flour or all-purpose flour	1 ½ cups
Hodgson Mill oat bran flour blend	½ cup
Dry yeast	1 package
Egg substitute	4 ounces
Warm water	2 ounces
Salt	1 teaspoon
Oil (canola is fine; walnut is special)	1 tablespoon
Honey	1 tablespoon

Knead and cycle through breadmaker as for white bread. The oat bran absorbs water slowly, so at first the dough should look wet and sticky. If it does, wait till later to do anything about it. Poke a finger into the dough when about 10 more minutes of the last kneading remain. If the dough seems tough and doesn't stick to your finger at all, add a tablespoon of water, let it mix a minute, and retest. If it's very sticky, add a tablespoon of flour, let it mix for a minute, and retest. Bake between light and medium; the egg makes it brown too much otherwise. After it's baked, do not cover it except loosely for the first 3 hours, so that the crust stays crispy.

This recipe makes about a1-pound loaf. The bread has about 0.7 gram fat per 1-ounce slice. Unlike a bakery's challah, it has no egg yolks, so it has no cholesterol.

Cinnamon Raisin Bread

Ingredient	Amount
Dry yeast	1 package
Bread flour	2 ¼ cups
Hodgson's Oat bran flour	¾ cup
Honey	1 tablespoon
Canola or walnut oil	1 tablespoon
Warm water	9 ounces
Salt or NuSalt	1 teaspoon
Raisins	¾ cup
Walnuts, crumbled	¼ cup
Optional additions:	
Granulated fructose	¼ cup
Ground cinnamon	2 teaspoons
Chinese five-spice	½ teaspoon

Put the first 7 ingredients (down to the Salt or NuSalt) in a breadmaker. Start the breadmaker's cycle of kneading as for white bread. The oat bran absorbs water slowly, so at first the dough should look wet and sticky. If it does, wait till later to do anything about it. Poke a finger into the dough when about 10 more minutes of the last kneading remain. If the dough seems tough and doesn't stick to your finger at all, add a tablespoon of water, let it mix a minute, and retest. If it's very sticky, add a tablespoon of flour, let it mix for a minute, and retest.

When 5 minutes remain in the last kneading, add the walnuts and raisins.

As soon as the second kneading ends, pull the dough out of the mixer. If it is too sticky to handle easily, add a teaspoon of bread flour here and there so you can grab it. If it is sticky at all, sprinkle flour onto the surface on which it will be rolled. Then spread it with a rolling pin to at least 9" x 12" on a flat surface (a cold marble surface resists the dough best). Cover with the sugar and spice mix. Roll up carefully, pressing to eliminate air pockets. Fold the loaf over once. Return it to the machine and let it rise, then bake to medium-light, so it stays moist and the raisins on the outside don't burn.

This recipe makes a two-pound loaf. For a coffee klatch, serve with buttercream icing (see Chapter 22).

Coffee Can Bread

A breadmaker provides one way to get around the uncertainties of making a successful yeast-dough bread from scratch. Another way is to make a batter bread. This one is especially good for breakfast because it has big, irregular nooks and crannies, just like an English muffin. My mom makes this soft, flavorful bread for me when I visit. The recipe makes two smallish loaves.

Ingredient	Amount
Flour	1 1/2 cups
Dry yeast	1 package
Warm water	1/2 cup
Nonfat milk	1/2 cup
Breadspread	1/2 cup
Grated parmesan cheese	2/3 cup
Optional substitute for cheese:	
Corn meal	1/3 cup
Salt or NuSalt	1 teaspoon
Egg substitute	4 ounces
Flour	2 cups

Combine the first amount of flour and the yeast in a ceramic or glass bowl. Heat the next 5 ingredients in a ceramic or glass bowl to 105° degrees (warmer than your finger but not hot). Pour over the flour and yeast. Beat until smooth. Add the egg substitute. Beat well. Add the last amount of flour. Mix until smooth.

Spray the insides of two 1-pound coffee cans with cooking spray (Pam brand or any other cooking oil that comes in a spray can). Add a tablespoon of corn meal to each can. Cover the cans with their plastic lids. Shake the corn meal around to cover the sides and bottom of the can. Remove the lids. Pour out any excess corn meal. Spoon the batter into the two cans equally. Cover loosely with wax paper. Let rise at 85° until the batter reaches near the top. Uncover and bake at 375° for 35 minutes. Put the cans low in the oven. Slide loaves out of cans when fresh from the oven. Cool 10 minutes before slicing.

Serve with breadspread (see Chapter 14). If you substituted corn meal for the cheese, the bread goes well with jams.

FOCACCIA

Making focaccia is rewarding, not only because fresh bread tastes wonderful but also because the investment in time is small and the results are much more predictable than when trying to make a loaf of bread from scratch.

Focaccia has to rise only about a quarter of an inch to be a success. As someone who has tried and usually failed to make a good loaf of bread from scratch, because it rose either too much or too little, focaccia is my kind of bread.

Serve it fresh; its great surface area makes it dry out easily. To take a portion, tear off a piece. Use where you would any chewy, crunchy bread. It's especially good with salads.

Focaccia freezes all right in a heavy-duty gallon-size plastic bag. Squeeze out all the air that you can before sealing the bag, or else the focaccia will dry badly. A frozen focaccia gives you a great head start on making a quick pizza. You can thaw it in about a minute in a microwave.

———

Focaccia (Pizza Bread) from Scratch by Hand

Ingredient	Amount
White flour	1 ½ cups
Warm water	½ cup
Dry yeast	1 package
Italian seasoning	½ teaspoon
Salt or NuSalt	½ teaspoon
Breadspread or olive oil	1 tablespoon
Honey	1 teaspoon
Optional for cheese-lovers:	
Decrease flour to	1 ¼ cup
Add finely grated low-fat or	
fat-free parmesan cheese	¼ cup

Put the dry ingredients in a bowl that holds at least a quart, and mix them a little. Add the warm water and the breadspread. Mix with a wooden spoon till it gets too hard to mix, about a minute. Then squash the mix together with your hands repeatedly. Add a tablespoon of flour at a time if the mix sticks to your fingers. Add a tablespoon of water if the mix won't stay stuck altogether in one lump. Keep squashing the mix together for 5 minutes. This makes the gluten in the flour stick together, forming a network that holds the water, the starch in the flour, and everything else. Then the yeast can make it rise without the bubbles popping out. Roll the dough into a ball and put it back in the bowl. Cover with a moist thin towel, put it in a warm place (e.g., on top of a refrigerator), and let it rise for 10 to 20 minutes until your topping is ready. Don't worry about the honey making the dough taste sweet. It won't. It's just there to insure that the dough will rise fast.

Let the dough rise for a few minutes until the ball is about twice as big around as after kneading. Pull the dough out of the bowl by hand, roll it into a ball, and, in midair, pull it out into the shape and size of a dish. If the dough sticks to your hands when you pull it out, it will stick to a roller and the pan. Don't let it.

Sprinkle a tablespoon of flour onto a 12-inch pizza pan. Lay the dough onto the floured pan. Spread another spoonful of flour over the top surface of the dough before and as you roll it, too. With a pizza rolling pin, a regular rolling pin, or the heels of your hands, roll or squash out the dough until it fills the pizza pan. Don't squash out the very edge. Leave a lip about 1/2-inch wide. This helps to keep the toppings on the pizza, and it helps keep the edge from burning before the rest of the pizza is baked enough. To use this as a thin pizza crust only, the dough is ready now to add toppings.

To make a focaccia, or if you like a thick-crust pizza, cover the crust with a dishtowel, and let it rise another 10 to 20 minutes. Cover the center third of the dough lightly with low-fat mozzarella. This is necessary to add weight so the foccacia doesn't turn into a giant ballooning pita. Bake for 5 to 10 minutes at 425° or until lightly browned. Bake this on a preheated pizza stone if you have one; it bakes faster, with a crunchier outside and a softer inside.

ALTERNATIVE #1: FOCACCIA OR PIZZA BREAD FROM THE BREADMAKER

Toss the above ingredients into a breadmaker, start the machine, and let it raise the dough for 10 to 20 minutes after the second kneading. If you prefer a thin crust, don't let the dough rise at all after the second kneading. If your breadmaker won't handle such a small amount of dough, increase the flour to 2 cups and the water to 2/3 cup. For a 12-inch pizza or focaccia, pinch off a quarter of the dough before you pull or roll it to fit the pan. By hand, roll the remnant into inch-thick breadsticks and bake them on an ungreased cookie sheet for about 5 minutes at 425° or until slightly browned. For a large pizza, use all of the dough.

ALTERNATIVE #2, PIZZA BREAD FROM THE GROCERY STORE

There are several brands of pizza bread available from the grocery store nowadays. They may have distressing amounts of garlic and onion in them, so be careful. I can't handle Boboli brand, for instance, but I can tolerate half or less of a "ZA" multigrain pizza bread.

If you want ready-made crust that's plain, get an uncut loaf of French or Italian bread, cut it lengthwise into slices as thick as you please, spread one side with a teaspoon of olive oil, and heat it in a preheated oven at 375° for about 5 minutes or until it just starts to brown a little.

PIZZA

This section is meant to give you some enjoyable alternatives to greasy crusts, saturated-fat cheeses, and fatty meat toppings. Go ahead, try them. Expand your horizons.

Smoky Vegetarian Pizza

Ingredient	Amount
12-inch pizza crust	(See previous recipes.)
Texas Sweet or Vidalia onion	$\frac{1}{8}$-inch slice (about $\frac{1}{4}$ cup, cut into large pieces)
Olive oil	1 teaspoon
Fresh basil leaves, chopped	1 tablespoon
Ground oregano	1 teaspoon or to taste
Asparagus	$\frac{1}{4}$ pound
Mushrooms	$\frac{1}{4}$ pound
Fresh tomato	$\frac{1}{4}$ pound
Smoked tofu	4 ounces
Fat-free mozzarella	4 ounces
Fat-free grated parmesan	2 tablespoons

Put the onion in a small saucepan. Add one teaspoon of olive oil and $\frac{1}{4}$ cup of water and bring to a boil. Let boil for about 5 minutes until the water steams away and the onion browns well. Watch it; don't let it blacken. Reduce heat to a simmer and add another $\frac{1}{4}$ cup of water. Let simmer for a couple of minutes until the onion looks gooey.

Preheat the oven to 475°. Chop the asparagus into pieces about $\frac{1}{2}$-inch to 1-inch long (shorter if it's thick, mature asparagus). Slice the mushrooms $\frac{1}{8}$- to $\frac{1}{16}$-inch thick. Chop the tomato into small bits so it will go far.

Spread the olive oil onto the crust, using your fingers. Sprinkle on the basil and oregano, erratically so that each bite will taste different. Spread the bits of onion and the raw veggies over the pizza. Doing so somewhat erratically is okay, but keep the overall thickness pretty uniform over the pizza so it will cook evenly.

Grate the smoked tofu and the mozzarella. Sprinkle both over the pizza. Add grated parmesan. Bake for 10 minutes at 475°, or until pizza crust starts to brown at the edges. After the first 7 minutes, spray the pizza 4 or 5 times with water from a spray bottle. This will help the mushrooms and asparagus to cook without drying.

Prefer a tart, moist pizza topping? Use dry cottage cheese instead of mozzarella or other cheeses. Fork or spoon it onto the pizza. Don't substitute regular cottage cheese; it releases too much water as it bakes.

Let the pizza cool slightly before slicing it.

Turkey-Artichoke White Pizza

Ingredient	Amount
Cooked turkey breast	4 ounces
Cara Mia artichoke hearts*	4 ounce jar
Broccoli stems	1 large (2–4 ounces)
Pizza crust	(See previous recipes.)
Italian seasoning	½ teaspoon
Corn starch	1 tablespoon
Water	4 ounces

Chop the turkey breast and the broccoli stems into small, bite-size pieces. Pour most of the oil off the top of the artichoke hearts and discard it. Pour off the rest of the liquid and save it in a small saucepan. Slice the artichoke hearts about ⅛-inch thick.

With your finger, mix the corn starch and water in a cup. Add the suspension to the liquid from the artichoke hearts in the saucepan. Stirring constantly, heat over medium heat just until the sauce comes to a boil and thickens. Let it cool a little. Stir it; if it's too thick to ladle onto the pizza easily, add another 2 ounces of water, heat to boiling again, and cool again.

Spread a teaspoon of olive oil on the pizza crust. Sprinkle on the Italian seasoning. Add the artichoke hearts, turkey, and broccoli bits. Cover all with sauce, a tablespoon at a time. Cover with low-fat mozzarella or dry cottage cheese. Bake for 10 minutes at 475°, or until the crust starts to brown at the edges. Cool slightly. Slice. Enjoy.

*Caution: Contains garlic.

No-Cheese Pizza

You can get much the same pizza at a restaurant, but the wait staff probably won't believe that you want it this way—without mozzarella. Try it, though, and you'll know why. Lay off the mozz, and you don't drown all the good flavors.

Ingredient: Pesto Sauce	Amount	Ingredient: Pizza	Amount
Pizza crust (See previous recipes.)			
Garlic cloves	6	Sundried tomatoes	4
Olive oil	1/4 cup	Hot water	1/2 cup
Freshly chopped basil leaves	1/4 cup	Mushrooms	4 ounces
Pine nuts or walnuts	1/2 tablespoon	Black olives	8
Coarsely grated parmesan	2 tablespoons	Feta cheese	4 ounces
Salt	1/4 teaspoon		Optional: Dry cottage cheese 4 ounces
Nonfat milk	4 tablespoons		

SUNDRIED TOMATOES: Put the tomatoes in a cup. Add 1/2 cup of hot (almost boiling) water. Let stand 30 minutes. Remove the tomatoes from the stock and slice them about 1/4 inch thick with kitchen shears.

PESTO SAUCE: With a sharp knife, peel the dry husks off the garlic cloves. Put the garlic and oil in a small saucer or glass casserole lid. Roast at 275° for 30 minutes with lots of air circulation in the room—exhaust fan on or windows open (roasting drives off the sulfur compounds mightily). Let cool. Smash the soft garlic cloves with a fork. Pull out any tough skins that remain. Pour the mix into a mortar. Add the basil leaves and nuts. Grind with a pestle till mostly mashed. Add the grated parmesan and salt. Grind till cheese is mostly mixed in. Add 1 tablespoon of milk; mix till pasty. Add another tablespoon of milk; mix till thick. Add the last two tablespoons of milk; stir till a uniform thick sauce. (You can use a small blender instead of a mortar and pestle.)

MUSHROOMS, OLIVES, FETA: Slice 1/8-inch thick. Chop the olives finely. Cut the feta into 1/2-inch bits.

ASSEMBLING THE PIZZA: Start with a thin pizza crust. Spread half the pesto sauce onto the crust. Cover with sundried tomatoes, mushrooms, and olives. Sprinkle the bits of feta around, not trying to make it cover every inch. Add the dry cottage cheese if you want a moister, cheesier pizza; it won't spoil the taste the way mozzarella does. (You can keep the rest of the pesto sauce refrigerated and tightly sealed for up to a week.)

Bake: Bake at 475° for 10 minutes or until the edges of the crust start to brown. Do not let the feta cheese brown. Cool slightly before cutting.

New England Boiled Pizza

No, the whole pizza isn't boiled. The sauce is, though. So it isn't just a joke.

Question: What could be more comforting than a comfort food like pizza? Two comfort dishes rolled into one, that's what. Just as in the recipe in Chapter 19 for a New England Boiled Dinner, you don't need the fat and salt of ham to enjoy the old-fashioned comforting taste.

Pizza Crust: (See previous recipes.)

Topping:

Turkey Canadian bacon (2–3 thick slices)	1/4 pound
Baked potato, cut into pieces the size and shape of short French fries	1 medium
Baby carrots, cut into quarters lengthwise	6
Stalk of celery, cut into 1/4-inch slices	1/2
Sweet or mild onion, chopped, presoaked in 1 cup hot water at least 10 minutes	1/4 cup
Pickling spice, ground coarsely	1/4 teaspoon
Hot water	1 cup

In a small casserole, put the turkey Canadian bacon slices, celery, carrots, chopped onion (drain first), pickling spice, and a cup of water. Heat to boiling. (If using a microwave, use High for about 4 minutes). Simmer 10 minutes (power setting 2 out of 10 if using the microwave). Pour off the hot water into another small casserole.

Put a tablespoon of cornstarch in a round-bottomed cup. Add two tablespoons of water. Mix with a finger till there are no lumps. Swirl a little so it doesn't settle, then pour the starch and water mix into the hot water from cooking the veggies. Heat on medium with constant stirring till the solution thickens into a gravy.

Spread the hunks of potato, carrot, celery, onion, and Canadian bacon around the pizza. Then pour the sauce over everything, to a 1/2-inch from the edges of the crust. Drizzle a tablespoon of olive oil over the pizza.

Bake at 425° for 20 to 25 minutes, until the edges of the crust brown and the top browns a little here and there. Take a big spatula, slide it under the pizza, and see if the bottom is browning slightly. When it is, take it out of the oven. Cut into slices with a big pair of scissors or kitchen shears. Serve.

Simple Bread Stuffing

Ingredient	Amount to Serve Two
Prepackaged unseasoned bread crumbs	6 ounces
Celery	1 large stalk or 2 small
Optional: Dried celery	1 tablespoon
Vegit®*	2 shakes
Sage	¼ teaspoon
Salt or NuSalt	¼ teaspoon or to taste
Breadspread	2 tablespoons
Hot water	1 cup (if you use fresh celery)
	1 ¼ cup (if you use dried celery)

PREPARATION: In a large bowl, mix all ingredients except water and breadspread.

In a 2-cup measuring cup, melt the breadspread in the hot water. Speed the process along by mixing with a fork. Put the dry ingredients into a small casserole. Starting at the outside edges so they don't burn, pour the water and breadspread mixture evenly onto the dry ingredients. Cover loosely with a glass lid or aluminum foil. If you want a browned top, don't cover it; instead, spray buttery-flavored cooking spray on top for about 5 seconds.

COOKING: Bake at 375° for 30 minutes.

*Caution: Vegit® contains some stomach offenders.

Chapter 18

$\mathcal{P}$ASTA DISHES

$\mathcal{B}$UYING PASTA

Even a food as wholesome as pasta still needs a label check. It may have whole eggs in it if it looks yellow. Whole eggs make restaurant pasta special, more flavorful and toothsome; and eggs may be used in the expensive pasta in the refrigerator compartment of the supermarket. Semolina flour, which looks a bit yellow, is not whole wheat, but it does contain more protein than regular white flour.

To avoid poisoning yourself on spoiled pasta, don't use outdated refrigerated pasta, and look carefully at unrefrigerated (dry) pasta before you cook it. It can molder.

Fancy shapes cost more, but I know of no reason to pay more for one brand of dry pasta than another. The consistency of the cooked product, the texture if you will, depends on the fact that the pasta was dry to begin with, not on the brand. The final result after cooking is a compromise. If it starts out dry, it's going to require much more cooking than the soft, refrigerated pasta, and that's going to make the outside of the noodle more soft than the inside.

$\mathcal{M}$AKING PASTA

If you have a pasta maker, please use it. No, not every time, just when your supply runs out. Supply? Yes, you can keep homemade pasta very well. Make it, then dry it for an hour on a rack until it doesn't stick together. Then take a handful (4–6 ounces), roll it together gently just enough to fit into a quart-size freezer bag, zip up the seal on the bag, and freeze. Typical pasta recipes like the one below make enough for about eight people, so unless you have a big gang to feed, you'll have plenty to freeze.

Plain Homemade Pasta

Ingredient	Amount
All-purpose unbleached flour	2 cups
Egg substitute	6 ounces (equivalent to 3 eggs)
Salt or salt substitute	1/8 teaspoon
Canola or olive oil	1 tablespoon

Using these ingredients, follow the directions that come with your pasta maker. Don't leave the pasta maker clean and pristine. Do dust it with flour before each operation, so the product doesn't stick to the machine. Also, dust the noodles with flour before you run them through the machine each time, and before you even consider laying one noodle on top of another.

If you didn't get directions with the pasta maker, or if they're in Italian and you don't read Italian, try the following. Start by making fettucine, not spaghetti; it's easier.

Mix all ingredients together just till they stick together and look uniform in color. Cut or pull the dough apart, into eight balls that are approximately equal in size. Run a ball through the pasta maker at its thickest setting. Fold over the product. Run it through the machine again. Do this several times until the noodle extrudes from the machine without shredding or balking. Do the same for all eight balls. Then, set the machine two notches tighter and process each noodle once. Tighten again by a couple of notches and reprocess. Do this until the needles are as thin as you want. For fettucine, a setting of 5 out of 7 on the classic Marcato Atlas hand-crank machine produces a full-bodied noodle. A setting of 6 out of 7 produces a thinnish noodle that holds more sauce and is easier to roll on a fork.

Fancy Homemade Pasta

Here are some additions, if you want pasta that's more tasty or colorful. Remember, though, that the pasta is the basic part of the recipe. If you are going to put something highly flavorful on it, use plain pasta. Spicy pasta is better used for plain dishes, in which you want to taste the pasta. An example of a simple pasta dish recipe follows the pasta cooking instructions.

TASTY, SPOTTED PASTA: Add 1 teaspoon ground oregano, or 1 teaspoon ground basil, or $\frac{1}{2}$ teaspoon of each.

ORANGE PASTA: Use tomatoes entirely instead of egg substitute.

GREEN PASTA: Use 3 ounces of pureed spinach (not chopped) and 3 ounces of egg substitute.

Pasta by Hand-Crank Machine: Using the Marcato Atlas Hand-Crank Pasta Maker

Put the flour and salt in a wide bowl. Add the egg substitute and oil on top, and work them in with a wooden spoon. As soon as the mixture holds together in one ball, dip it into loose flour and run it through the pasta maker on the thickest-rolling setting. The secret of making pasta without it sticking together is continuing to spread a little flour onto the surface before each pass through the rollers.

Fold the dough over once, onto itself, and pass it through the rollers. Repeat this process until the dough does not stick to the rollers at all and makes a uniform, uncracked sheet. If it's too dry, still breaking apart after half a dozen foldings and rollings, add another tablespoon of water, knead it in slowly, and start rolling again. As soon as it rolls through the maker without breaking up, it's kneaded enough.

Divide the dough into eighths. Increase the fineness setting on the pasta maker by a notch and reroll the pieces of dough. Then increase by two notches at a time until you get the thinness that you want. Don't try making angel hair the first time; it's too difficult.

COOKING PASTA

Boil a quart of water for every eighth of the pasta that you cook. Add $\frac{1}{2}$ teaspoon of salt or salt substitute and a teaspoon of oil for each quart of water. Drop no more than one handful of pasta at a time into the boiling water. This stuff cooks fast. When fresh, it needs no more than 2 minutes, but cooking for up to 5 minutes may not make it too soft. When frozen for a few weeks, it may take longer, 5 minutes or more, depending on how firm you like it.

Fettucine al Burro

Ingredient	Amount to Serve 2
Homemade fettucine	6 ounces
Hot water	1 quart
Salt or salt substitute	1/2 teaspoon
Canola or olive oil	1 teaspoon
Breadspread	4 ounces
Nonfat sour cream	2 ounces
Olive oil	1 tablespoon
Weight Watchers grated parmesan cheese	1 tablespoon or to taste

Mix the breadspread, sour cream, and tablespoon of olive oil together in a small bowl. Put the hot water, salt, and teaspoon of oil into a kettle. Heat to boiling. Add the fettucine. Cook as above until as done as you like it. Drain fettucine in a colander. Rinse with hot water.

Put the fettucine into a bowl. Add the breadspread, sour cream, and olive oil mix. Toss to coat the pasta evenly. Sprinkle grated cheese on top. Garnish with parsley, basil, or oregano as desired. Serve.

Fettucine Carbonara

In the original form, fettucine carbonara is a salty, spicy dish, dripping with egg and cream sauce. See if you don't agree that this version has as much creaminess and taste as you want.

Ingredient	Amount to Serve 2
Fettucine	4 ounces
Hot water	1 quart
Salt or salt substitute	1/2 teaspoon
Chopped green onion	1/4 cup, with 6 inches of greens, presoaked in hot water for at least 10 minutes
Buttery-flavor cooking spray	
Cool water	4 ounces
Turkey ham	2 ounces
Nonfat sour cream	4 ounces
Grated parmesan cheese	2 tablespoons

Eggbeaters or other egg substitute	2 ounces (equivalent to one egg)
Olive oil	1 teaspoon
Oregano, crushed leaf	1/2 teaspoon

Cut up the turkey ham into long, thin slices about the size of a half-strip of bacon after it's cooked. If you are going to add veggies, clean and cut them up now.

Measure out 1/2 teaspoon of oregano into a mortar. Grind it with a pestle until it's finely ground.

Put hot water and salt into the pasta pot. Put the pasta pot on to boil. When it comes to a rolling boil, add the fettucine and stir every minute or two to keep the fettucine from sticking together. As soon as the mixture comes to a boil again, start the sauce.

Spray a small saucepan with buttery-flavor cooking spray for 3 seconds. Put the chopped knob onion into the pan. Add 2 ounces of cool water and bring to a fast boil on medium-high heat. Let all the water boil away and continue heating until the onions are half-browned. Immediately add another 2 ounces of cool water and the ham.

When the sauce comes to a boil, either add veggies and let them steam for 2 to 3 minutes or, if you're making this the simpler way, go right to completing the sauce. For this, remove the saucepan from heat. Then add the nonfat sour cream, the low-fat grated parmesan cheese, and the egg substitute. Stir gently with a teaspoon or other smallish spoon until the sauce is smooth and uniformly thin. Put it back on the heat at medium and stir constantly until it thickens but does not boil (takes only a minute or two).

As soon as the fettucine is no longer tough to the tooth, pour it into a colander, rinse it, and divide the cooked fettucine into two warmed pasta bowls. Add 1/2 teaspoon of olive oil to each portion and toss for a few seconds.

Sprinkle the ground oregano onto the pasta. Ladle the sauce on top. Serve with some white grape juice or sparkling apple juice.

This does not make a balanced meal without a salad unless you add vegetables. Here is a suggestion to add some plant life to your carbonara. Take a whole portobello mushroom and 1/4 pound each of French-cut green beans (sliced the long way), pea pods, and broccoli stems sliced into shoestring potato shapes. Use equal amounts of these vegetables so no one taste overpowers the rest of the dish. Simmer all veggies for 2 minutes in the small saucepan before adding the egg substitute and sour cream. The portobello mushroom makes an especially good addition, but it has one drawback: The sauce comes out gray instead of creamy yellow-tan.

Turkey and Pasta

Ingredient	Amount
Turkey breast, sliced	3 ounces
Savory	pinch
Broth, chicken or turkey	5 tablespoons
Nonfat sour cream	2 tablespoons
Bite-size pasta	3 ounces
Cranberry sauce	2 ounces

Stir the first four ingredients together. Heat together slowly till hot but not bubbling or boiling.

Meanwhile, boil the pasta in a pint of salted water till al dente. Drain. Add the cranberry sauce. Mix it with the pasta. Reheat the pasta and cranberry mixture till hot.

Serve turkey mix on the side of the pasta and cranberry combo. A baked yam is okay with this. A green vegetable would add more contrast of flavor and color.

Chicken Stroganoff

Why do onions cause us such distress? How can we get the oniony taste we enjoy with meat, and avoid the aftereffects? Onions contain organic sulfur compounds. When subjected to the acid in the stomach, these compounds are broken down to form sulfuric acid. That's right: battery acid in your stomach. No wonder it hurts! But you don't have to swallow the battery acid to get the taste of onions. Leeks have a moderate amount of the onion-tasty stuff and little of the acid-forming stuff. And, by browning them strategically, you get a double effect: more flavor and even less acid. The organic sulfur compounds are volatile and are dissipated fast by heating to high temperature and chasing them away with steam.

Ingredient	Amount to Serve 2
Bite-size pasta—fusilli, shells, macaroni, rotelli, or wide soup noodles	6 ounces
Hot water	2 quarts
Salt or NuSalt	
Olive oil	1 teaspoon
Leek (or knob [green] onion)	½, including the first 6" of greens

Tough green leek or onion tops	2–3" lengths for garnish
Buttery-flavor cooking oil spray	
Cool water	1/2 cup
Fresh mushrooms	6 ounces
Chicken bouillon granules	1 teaspoon
Nonfat sour cream	6 ounces
Grilled chicken breast	1
Pepper from a mill that grinds finely	1/8 teaspoon

Tools
Five-quart kettle
One-quart saucepan
Wide-blade chopping knife
Cutting board

PREPARATION

If you don't have a leftover grilled chicken breast, spread a teaspoon of plain yogurt on a skinless chicken breast (need not be boneless) and broil in a toaster oven for 15 to 20 minutes, turning once, until done (no pink remains when you poke a sharp knife down to the middle and peek). If the chicken breast is bone-in, peel the bones off the breast after it cools a bit.

Cut the leek into coins 1/8- to 1/4-inch thick, and chop the coins in half. Leeks are so mild that you don't have to do this under water (it's hard to cut vegetables with a diver's helmet on, anyway). Slice the mushrooms 1/8- to 1/4-inch thick. Cut the chicken into chunks about 1 inch by 1 inch by 1/4 inch.

COOKING

Put the kettle on a burner at medium high with 2 quarts of water, the salt, and the oil in it.

As soon as the water starts cooking, coat the inside of the saucepan lightly with cooking oil spray. Put the pan on medium heat and add the chopped leek. Add 1/4 cup of water after a few seconds and cook a couple of minutes until the water is all gone. While it's cooking, shake the pan by the handle once in a while to spread the leek evenly over the pan and separate the bigger hunks into little pieces. Keep watching the pan, because as soon as the water is all gone and the leek starts to brown nicely, you must add another 1/4 cup of water and remove immediately from the heat. That's so the leeks give off all their acid into the air and develop a good taste, but get quenched from burning.

With the water in the kettle at a rolling boil, add the pasta. Go ahead with the rest of the preparation of the sauce as you occasionally stir the pasta and sample it. Cook the pasta 8 to 10 minutes until it's as soft (all the way through) as you like it. Then immediately turn off the heat and take the kettle off the burner. When the stroganoff is done, drain off the water from the noodles by pouring all through a colander. Rinse once with hot tap water before serving.

To the browned leeks and water, add the bouillon granules. Swirl the pan lightly until the granules dissolve. Add the mushrooms, cover the pan, and simmer for 3 minutes or until the mushrooms start to darken slightly.

Reduce the heat to low. Add the sour cream and the chicken. Stir a few seconds with a small ladle until the color is even and the mix is as thick as a gravy. Do **not** let the sauce boil, or it won't stay smooth.

COOKING

On plates heated for 5 minutes in a 150° oven, put servings of noodles. Ladle stroganoff on top, leaving a margin of noodles for color and texture contrast. A few sprigs of leek greens make a nice garnish and add a nice aroma, without putting acid into your stomach.

Mushrooms Stroganoff

Prepare and cook as for Chicken Stroganoff, with two changes: Eliminate the chicken, and use 8 ounces of portobello mushrooms instead of 6 ounces of smaller mushrooms. Slice the mushrooms about 1/4-inch thick. All the cooking they need is to be sauteed in a teaspoon of olive oil and 2 tablespoons of water for 1 to 2 minutes, or until they begin to soften.

Chapter 19

$\mathcal{P}$OTATOES AND POTATO-BASED DISHES

$\mathcal{P}$otatoes can always be baked or boiled. The smaller you cut the pieces, the faster they cook. If you think it a waste of time and electrical energy cooking potatoes in a pot of water, and have no worries about what microwaving does to the nutrition content of your foods, then microwave your potatoes. There's no telling what will be revealed in the future, but a few Russian findings have surfaced suggesting that microwaving lowers vitamin content, can twist food molecules into carcinogens, and lowers the "vital energy field content," whatever that is. A literature search I performed did not subtantiate any of these claims.

If you opt for microwaving, follow your oven's directions, and you'll almost always get satisfactory results. There are a number of things the books don't tell you, however. One is about water content. Idaho potatoes can have as much as 65 percent dry weight. New red potatoes have only about a third of that. Since it's the water molecules in the food that the microwaves set to jumping (heating, that is), you might think the red potatoes will cook slower because they have more water to heat. Wrong. They take less time. Also, because they are mostly water, they won't microwave cook into baked potatoes. They'll microwave cook into something like half-dry boiled potatoes.

Idaho potatoes are odd eating straight out of the microwave too. Because they cook by steaming themselves from the inside, their skins inevitably get damp from the inside. This is acceptable if you don't eat the skins and don't want much taste, but the insides will lack the taste of a browned potato skin. The recipes to follow cope with both types of potato and produce old-fashioned, tasty results.

Boiled Red Potatoes Fast and Easy

Ingredient	Amount to Serve 2
Red potatoes	1 pound
Warm water	2 ounces
Breadspread	1 tablespoon
Parsley or dill	1 teaspoon
Optional for tougher stomachs:	
Sweet Hungarian paprika	$1/4$ teaspoon
or Vegit®*	$1/4$ teaspoon

Tub and scrub a pound of potatoes. New potatoes, golf-ball size or smaller, should be cooked whole. Bigger reds should be quartered so they cook evenly. Put the potatoes into a saucepan, (glass or ceramic casserole for 'waving), add almost enough water to float them (or $1/4$ cup of water if microwaving), and cover loosely. Boil about 10 minutes until the taters soften, or 'wave on high for 7-10 minutes. Let stand a minute. Wearing a potholder mitt, remove the lid quickly so no steam gets you. Stab a piece of potato with a fork. It should break easily. If it doesn't, check the water supply in the bottom, add a tablespoon if it's dry, and cook for additional 1-minute increments until the potatoes pass the fork test.

When the potatoes are cooked, add the breadspread and your choice of parsley or dill. With a tablespoon, roll the potatoes in the liquid and the herb until well coated.

If you prefer brown, zestier potatoes and your stomach can handle a little onion, skip the herbs and add the paprika and Vegit before you roll the potatoes to coat them. The potatoes can be served hot or cold. If you plan to serve them cold, do so the same day or the next, not later. Potatoes don't keep well. They get that leftover potato off-taste. And please don't reheat them, or they'll get that leftover taste for sure.

*Caution: Vegit® contains some stomach offenders.

Quick Baked Idaho (Russet) Potatoes

Tub 'em and scrub 'em. A Scrunge works better than cloth. Cut out the eyes and the bruises. Pierce them down to the center. Do this in two places for medium potatoes (one through-and-through jab is fine as long as you make it on a cutting board, not holding the potato in midair), and in three or four places for jumbos so they don't crack or explode. If you've had to trim out any big holes, don't add more holes (the potatoes dry too much), just pierce down to the center from the site of trimming.

Put the potatoes on a dish that will withstand microwaving. Corelle works fine, and so should most stoneware *as long as it has no metallic trim* (gold, silver, etc.). If you are cooking three or more potatoes, arrange them in a small ring around the center of the plate. Their long ends should face each other but not touch. A quarter-inch separation is enough, despite what the books say. Put the dish of potatoes in the center of the floor of the microwave.

Microwave on High for 2 minutes for one potato, 3 minutes for two potatoes, 4 minutes for three potatoes, or 5 minutes for four potatoes. Tap any small potatoes with the bottom of a tablespoon (okay, you can use your finger if you're tough and won't sue me if you get burned). If they indent, they're done; pull them out. Wearing a potholder mitt, turn the potatoes that are still tough. Twist them around 180° on their long axis so the down side is up.

Microwave for the same length of time less a minute for each potato removed. All potatoes should now pass the spoon test. Don't stop cooking on this note. Put the potatoes into a toaster oven, well-separated but all directly under the cooking element. Brown them slightly by toasting at the toaster setting of Dark. If your oven doesn't do that, it's just as good to preheat it to 450° while the potatoes are microwaving, then heat for 3 to 5 minutes. Remove the browned potatoes from the toaster oven carefully, because the skins are now extremely hot.

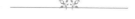

French "Fries"

Imagine it: real french fries, their outsides brown and saturated with oil, then smothered in ketchup. Yum. Enough to give you heartburn just thinking about it. But here's a recipe that gives you more than just an acceptable substitute. This combination is 3+ Mmm on a scale of 0 to 4 Mmms.

Ingredient	Amount to Serve 2
Idaho potatoes, about 6 ounces each	2 medium
Egg Beaters	1–2 ounces
Sweet Hungarian paprika	$1/4$–$1/2$ teaspoon
Buttery-flavor cooking spray	
Genuine Sun Brand tomato chutney, to dip	
Salt or NuSalt to taste	

Cut the potatoes into strips no more than $3/8$-inch square in cross-section. Dry them with a paper towel. Put them in a shallow bowl. Dust them with the paprika. Pour the egg substitute over them. Toss with your fingers to coat them evenly. Spray generously (for about 5 to 8 seconds) a 6-inch by 9-inch baking pan with the butter-flavor cooking spray. Arrange the potatoes in the pan so they don't touch each other much.

Bake in a preheated toaster oven at 425° for 20 to 25 minutes, until golden brown. Serve with ½ teaspoon of the chutney or breadspread (see Chapter 14).

Half-Hour New England Boiled Dinner

You don't need all the fat and salt of ham to enjoy the smoky taste of a New England boiled dinner. Turkey Canadian bacon is only 5 percent fat. Sliced, it imparts the smoked taste to the vegetables quickly.

Ingredient	Amount
Turkey Canadian bacon	½ pound (6 thick slices)
Medium potatoes, peeled and cut in quarters	4–5
Yam, peeled and cut into 12 pieces	1 large
Whole baby carrots	½ pound
White knob onion, chopped in ¼-inch slices	¼ cup
Pickling spice	1 teaspoon
Water to half-fill a	2-quart casserole dish

Line the bottom of the casserole dish with the turkey Canadian bacon slices. Over them layer yams, potatoes, and carrots, then sprinkle on the chopped onion and the pickling spice. Add water to cover the potatoes but not the carrots or onions. Heat to boiling (on High in the microwave, about 4 minutes per pound or 15 minutes total). Simmer for 15 minutes (2 out of 10 in the microwave) or until a fork goes through the potatoes and yams easily. A-yep, you can serve it now.

Salmon Dip

Ingredient	Amount
Salmon steak	½ pound
Nonfat plain yogurt	1 tablespoon

Rosemary	1 teaspoon
Tarragon	1 teaspoon
Nonfat sour cream	8 ounces
Salt or NuSalt	$1/2$ teaspoon

Place salmon in a shallow baking pan. Cover with half of the rosemary and tarragon. Spread yogurt over the spices. Broil salmon for about 15 minutes until light pink all the way through. Let cool. Remove the bone and skin, and mash the meat with a fork. In a 1-quart sealable plastic container, combine the salmon, the sour cream, the remainder of the rosemary and tarragon, and the salt. Chill. Can be used as a dip with crackers.

Hot Salmon Spread and Hash Browns

Make hash-browned potatoes as in Chapter 14. Separate hash browns into four patties. Top each patty with $1/4$ cup salmon dip. Warm in microwave or broiler oven just until dip is warm. Serve immediately.

Irish Stir-Fry

What do you call a dish that's a stir-fry without rice or noodles? It's certainly not Chinese. On the other hand, would you believe that soy and ginger go nicely with potatoes? This is another fast dish that needs little or nothing to make it a complete meal. Check the serving suggestions at the end of the recipe for side dishes that work well.

Ingredient	Amount
Baking potatoes	2 medium
Cauliflower florets	3 ounces
Celery	1 stalk
Carrot	1 large, 2 small, or 6 baby carrots
Mushrooms	2 ounces
Chicken breast, skinless	1
Low-acid onion (Vidalia), chopped and presoaked for 10 minutes in hot water	$1/4$ cup
Apple cider vinegar	1 tablespoon
Low-salt soy sauce	1 teaspoon

Bragg Liquid Aminos	2 teaspoons
Powdered ginger	1/4 teaspoon
Vegit®*	1/2 teaspoon
Flour	2 tablespoons
Canola oil	2 tablespoons

Scrub the potatoes. Dice into a saucepan and boil till tender (about 10 minutes); or pierce each one twice to let steam out, and microwave for 4 to 5 minutes until softened. Let cool until they can be handled without burning you. Meantime, wash the chicken breast and slice it 1/4-inch thick, then set it aside. Chop the carrots and celery into bite-size pieces no more than 1/4-inch thick. Cut the mushrooms into 1/4-inch thick pieces and set aside.

Put 1 tablespoon of canola oil into a wok or 12-inch skillet. Heat until oil thins but does not smoke. Drain the chopped onions and add them to the hot pan. Saute on medium until the onions brown slightly. Coat the chicken pieces by shaking 2 tablespoons of flour onto them. Saute, stirring and turning occasionally, for 2 to 3 minutes until chicken pieces are browned slightly and have turned white all the way through. Remove chicken and onions from pan.

Add 1 tablespoon of canola oil to the pan. Dump in the celery, carrots, and cauliflower. Stir-fry for a minute. Add one cup of hot water. Add the apple cider vinegar, Vegit, and ginger. Stir to bring up the brown, chickeny stuff stuck on the bottom of the pan. Cover the pan. Let boil for 3 minutes. As it does, cut the microwave-baked potatoes into hunks about 1/2-inch by 1/2-inch by 1-inch thick.

Add the mushrooms to the pan. Stir. Boil another minute. Add the chicken and cut-up potatoes. Bring to a boil again. Stir to coat the chicken and potatoes with the gravy that has formed. Transfer to a serving bowl. Serve.

SERVING SUGGESTIONS: A sweet potato makes a good side dish. Crusty bread sops up the juices nicely. Homemade cranberry sauce (see index) makes a wonderful contrast.

*Caution: Vegit® contains some stomach offenders.

Chapter 20

$\mathcal{R}$ICE AND RICE-BASED DISHES

White Rice

Chinese people would think Minute Rice is a crazy idea. To them, white rice is not supposed to be flaky, each grain separate. It's supposed to be sticky, so it can be eaten with chopsticks. It's easy enough to serve this way, too. Just be sure to use a sharpish-bladed serving spoon, not a dull, thick spoon, so you can scoop the amount that you want.

Here's another good reason to use white rice that's not precooked: It's fast. There's no reason it should take longer to cook than the rest of the meal.

There's a big reason not to serve white rice, though. It is absorbed about as fast as pure sugar, so it makes you feel hungry again fast and stresses your insulin output. My advice is to cook brown rice instead. But if you want white, here's how to make it.

Ingredient	Amount to Serve 2
White rice	4 ounces
Hot water	8 ounces

Put the two ingredients into a saucepan (glass or ceramic casserole if microwaving) that holds at least a quart. Cover completely but loosely. A Corelle plate works fine on a round casserole. (Remember, no metal in the microwave.) Heat the rice and water until it comes to a boil (in microwave on High for two minutes). Turn down the heat on your range to low, or if 'waving, stop it then so the pot doesn't boil over (sticky mess in microwave, casserole glued to floor of microwave, lid glued to casserole). Simmer for 10 minutes (microwave on the lowest setting that makes the rice water boil for a little while each minute; set at 1 or 2 out of 10).

You can serve immediately, as this simmering technique limits the live steam when you open the lid. It's safer to wait 1 to 5 minutes, and the rice will stay plenty hot in the microwave. Then serve it in the casserole so it stays hot at the table.

Brown or Wild Rice

Brown rice is the form of the grain that is absorbed more slowly and brings along more goodies such as protein, fiber, vitamins, and nutty flavor.

Ingredient	Amount to Serve 2
Brown, wild, or mixed rice	4 ounces
Hot water	6 ounces for chewy rice, up to 8 for soft

Additions to Jazz It Up

Before cooking:

Chicken or beef bouillon crystals	1 teaspoon
Celery, chopped finely	1 tablespoon

Before serving:

Slivered almonds 1 tablespoon

Put the rice and water into a saucepan (glass or ceramic casserole for 'waving) that holds at least a quart. Cover completely, but loosely. Heat to boiling (in microwave on High for 2 to 3 minutes). Turn down the range setting to simmer or stop the microwaving then so the pot doesn't boil over. Then simmer (microwave for 20 minutes on Low setting, 2 out of 10). Wearing hot-pad mitts, tip the pan slightly after 20 minutes to see if all the water is taken up. If not, continue another 2 to 5 minutes until no water remains in the bottom.

Wild rice may be too chewy for you unless you add another 4 ounces of boiling-hot water now and simmer for another 10 minutes or so.

You can serve this immediately, but if you have 'waved, watch for live steam burns when you open the lid. Better to wait 1 to 5 minutes, then serve.

Easy Mushroom Risotto

"The yuppie food of the '90's" is how risotto has been billed. On the other hand, the usual recipes for making it require half an hour of stirring. That makes for a very un-yuppie-like level of hard work in the kitchen. See if you find this version more reasonable.

Ingredient	Amount to Serve 2
Risotto rice (see below)	5 ounces
Porcini mushrooms	¼ ounce dry
Hot water	2 cups

Vegit®*	¼ teaspoon
Olive oil	1 tablespoon
Breadspread	1 teaspoon

Risotto is supposed to require a special Italian risotto rice, arborio preferably. A Spanish paella rice works too. If you want risotto and don't have any of this, there's no reason why you can't substitute any medium-grain rice. Unlike long-grained rice, all of these rices release much of their starch content into the cooking water, so it gets as thick as gravy. Why not? That's all gravy is anyway—water, flavoring, and enough starch to make a runny gel, plus a little fat to improve taste and the feel on the tongue. If you use medium-grain white rice, expect it to cook faster, because its grain is smaller than risotto rice, and expect it to be soft rather than al dente in the middle.

Break up the dry mushrooms, and put them into a cup of hot water to get them rehydrating. Put the olive oil into a range-safe ceramic saucepan. Heat on medium until it's hot. Add the rice and then the breadspread. Stir every few seconds, using a flat spatula, until the rice begins cracking or a few grains brown. Don't let it all get brown. The process should take only about 2 minutes.

Then, pour the mushrooms and water into the saucepan and add another cup of hot water. Add the Vegit and salt or salt substitute. Give it a few stirs until it's an even color. When it comes back to a boil, cover loosely and start simmering (or pop it into the microwave). Simmer (or 'wave on 2/10 maximum) for 13 minutes or until most of the liquid is taken up.

Sample the rice: Transfer a tad, maybe ¼ teaspoon, from the stirring spatula to a cold tablespoon, wait a few seconds, then taste it. The rice is cooked enough if it's al dente, just a little chewy on the inside.

Remove the risotto from the heat as soon as it is al dente. Stir in a couple of ice cubes to cool the sauce just a little. This helps keep the rice from soaking up all the sauce. Otherwise, it congeals as it stands. Serve it uncovered immediately, before it gets too thick.

*Caution: Vegit® contains some stomach offenders.

Rice Erroneous

This imitation of Rice-a-Roni is easy and adds flavor to all kinds of dinners.

Ingredient	**Amount to Serve 4 to 6**
Orzo or vermicelli (thin spaghetti) broken into short lengths (1" or less)	½ cup

Long-grain white rice (or parboiled brown rice)	1 cup
Chicken bouillon crystals	1 teaspoon
Dried celery	1 teaspoon
or chopped fresh celery	2 tablespoons
Vegit®*	½ teaspoon
or dried onion flakes if tolerated	1 teaspoon
Dried oregano	¼ teaspoon
or home-dried oregano leaves	1 teaspoon
Canola oil	1 tablespoon

Brown orzo or spaghetti lightly in oil in a 2-quart saucepan. Stir occasionally for 3 to 5 minutes until the pasta is golden brown, not blackened. Add 3 cups of hot water and all the other ingredients. Bring to a boil. Simmer, covered, about 15 minutes or until the water has been taken up by the rice and pasta.

*Caution: Vegit® contains some stomach offenders.

Hearty Greens and Tasty Rice
(30 to 45 Minutes Cooking Time)

Ingredient	Amount to Serve		
	1	**2**	**4**
Greens			
Fresh spinach, pounds	¼	½	1
Medium zucchini	½	1	2
Oregano, teaspoons	¼	½	1
Thyme, teaspoons	¼	½	1
Olive oil, tablespoons	1	2	4
Crumbled walnuts, tablespoons	1	2	4
Chutney: tomato or your choice	-- to taste --		
Saucepan size, quarts	1	1	2 or bigger
Rice			
Lundberg brown and wild rice mix, ounces	1	2	4
Dry lentils, ounces	1	2	4
Brown rice, ounces	1	2	4
Canola oil, tablespoons	½	1	2

Hot water, cups	³/₄	1 ½	3
Salt or NuSalt, teaspoons	¼	½	1
Glass or ceramic pot size, quarts	1	1	2
Approximate time to boil, minutes	1 ½	3	6

COOKING

Rice mix. Measure both kinds of rice and the lentils into a glass or ceramic pot. Pick through it with a fork, looking for stones. Discard any foreign matter. Rinse the mix with a potful of hot water. Pour off the water but don't drain—leave it good and wet. Add the hot water, oil, and salt. Cover tightly. Heat on medium-high on the range (or microwave on high) till it starts to boil. Simmer (or microwave at lowest setting) for 30 to 40 minutes, until all the water is taken up and the lentils sit on top looking fluffy.

Greens. When the rice mix has just begun simmering, take a semi-dull paring knife to the zucchini. With the knife edge down, as if you're ready to chop the zucchini in half, scrape the outside of the zucchini here and there as needed to remove any scars and bruises. Don't remove any of the healthy-looking dark green skin. Then get a potato peeler and whittle the zucchini just like a stick. Hold the zucchini at one end and slap the peeler along the rest of the length, to peel off thin slices that look like fettucine with a dark green border. Whittle onto a breadboard to save the peels. When you get down to seeds, turn the zucchini a tad so you can keep peeling off the goodie and leaving the baddie. If you're cooking for more than one, when you're left with an obscene-looking seedy end, don't cut it off. Instead, grab that end and start whittling the other half.

Spinach is grown in dirt, and it's got wraparound stems that hold the dirt tightly. So step one in cleaning is to get rid of the main source of the dirt. Pick up a bunch of leaves with your left hand, keeping the stems down. Grab all of the length of the stems with your right hand. Twist your wrists as if you're going to break a candy bar in halves to share with a buddy. Share the stems with your buddy the compost bucket.

Holding a couple of leaves at a time under warm or cool running water, slide your fingers over the spinach. Any transparent or slimy spinach has to go join your buddy. Leave the spinach nice and wet on a bread board.

Now pour the olive oil into a nonstick saucepan or wok. Slosh the oil around gently to coat the pan or wok. Now start heating the pan at medium heat on the range—use the 250° setting if you're using an electric wok. As soon as the pan starts getting hot, add the zucchini. When it starts to boil, add the spinach on top. After a minute, stir the spinach down into the hot zucchini. If your range is electric, immediately turn off the heat. If it's gas, wait half a minute, then turn off the heat.

SERVING

Place servings of hot vegetables and hot rice mix in a hot pasta bowl. Sprinkle crumbled walnuts on the rice. Add a garnish (see below). Put it at the 12 o'clock spot on the pasta bowl, and if some of it sticks out of the lip of the bowl, so much the better for looks.

Garnishes. The easiest is chutney. A little is just the touch to add zip to the rice mix. Find one that you savor but that doesn't attack your stomach with hotness. Sun brand tomato chutney is a favorite of mine. A big strawberry on a reserved uncooked spinach leaf looks great and refreshes the palate between bites of the hot stuff. Or add a big slice of lemon and a sprig of parsley. Somehow, lemon juice makes spinach both buttery and rousing enough to make you wanna growl like Popeye. Don't growl if you're eating with sensitive people, unless you follow it with a graceful little "A-yuk-yuk-yuk-yuk" as Popeye does.

Un-Garian Lecso

This started as a Hungarian dish. Before you say, "Uh, oh, ethnic food. . .weird stuff," let me inform you that Hungarian cuisine derived many of its techniques from the French. Some transfer vice versa has occurred, too. It was the Hungarians, not the French, who invented the croissant. The crescent shape was to celebrate a great military victory over the Turks. Nothing like biting the enemy's favorite symbol in half for breakfast, eh? Of course, when the French and Austrian victors took over from the Turks, they, in turn, occupied Hungary, but at least they were relatively benign overlords.

The authentic version of lecso (say letch'-o) is chock full of green peppers (from which comes the name), onions, and tomatoes. The tomatoes may have come from the influence of an Italian queen who moved into the palace with her Italian cooks in the Middle Ages. But lecso may have actually begun in Serbia, so let's forget about the genealogy and get to the cooking.

Authentic lecso has a tablespoon of Hungarian paprika per serving (yes, a tablespoon, not a teaspoon). When meat, usually veal and beef, is added, it's supposed to be called lecso with meat. Okay, your stomach wouldn't touch this conglomeration with a 10-foot spoon. But remember: A little of the more benign seasonings in this dish won't hurt you. And your palate has been sensitized to enjoy more delicate tastes because you've been laying off the offending foods.

Try this lecso just once and you may want to join those big, strapping veterans in the army of the Hapsburgs in toasting, "Magyar ember!" ("To the Hungarian man!").

Ingredient	Amount to Serve 2
White rice or parboiled brown rice	4 ounces
Hot water	8 ounces
Knob onion or leek	half, chopped coarsely, presoaked if possible
Buttery-flavor cooking spray	
Cool water	4 ounces
Skinless chicken breast	1
Turkey ham in a thick slice	2 ounces
Baby carrots, chopped into rounds	5, weighing 1 ounce
Cauliflower, broken into florets	1/4 quarter head, weighing 8 ounces
Plum tomatoes	2, cut into 6 slices each
Beef bouillon crystals	1 teaspoon
Hungarian sweet (not hot) paprika	1/2 teaspoon

Wash the vegetables. Slice the onion (or leek), the carrots, and the tomatoes. Break the cauliflower into florets.

Start the rice first. In a 1- to 2-quart glass or ceramic casserole (Pyrex or Corningware are best to heat fast and minimize sticking), put 8 ounces of hot water and the rice. Bring to a boil on the range and simmer 10 minutes (or use the microwave for 2:22 on HIGH then 10:00 on low (setting 2 on a scale of 1 to 10).

Spray the bottom of a 2-quart saucepan with buttery-flavor cooking spray for 3 seconds. Start heating the saucepan on medium-high. Add the onion (or leek). Add 2 ounces of cool water. Let boil till the water dries and half the onion gets tan or brown (not black). Add the next 2 ounces of cool water immediately, and the chicken and turkey ham. Let cook until the water is about gone and the meat has browned on one side. Add the vegetables, another 4 ounces of water, the bouillon crystals and the paprika. When the liquid comes to a boil, cover the pot and turn the heat down to Low. Simmer for 6 minutes or until the cauliflower can be pierced easily with a sharp nylon fork. Remove from heat. This dish will stay hot enough if it stands covered for 5 minutes or longer, as needed for the rice to finish cooking.

To serve, ladle the lecso over the rice. Serve with crusty bread and breadspread. The Magyars serve this with red wine; Knudsen concord grape juice has enough bite to substitute.

A Chinese Menu of Easy Stir-Fried Meat and Vegetable Recipes

Chinese food is fun. The preparation calls for cleaning and artful whacking, but little else. The cooking is quick. The eating is easy, requiring nary a knife. There is great variety in it, even surprises, in the textures, colors, and shapes. So keep it fun by not bending over backward to follow any one recipe slavishly.

The lists of ingredients below are, fittingly, a "Chinese menu" of alternatives. The directions are generalized to serve as many people as you wish and to make dozens of different combinations. First try the top suggestion in each category, unless you don't have it on hand. Remember, you don't have to go out and buy a dozen different exotic ingredients to do this "right." From each category of alternatives, just use the ingredient(s) that you like. This, even more than politics, is the art of the possible.

You can even throw out the idea of variety and just put one main vegetable into the dish, perhaps with a little meat and something crunchy to make a main dish of it. This restraint in variety can work very well if your main vegetable is fresh and if you make a flavorful sauce to go with it. If you try this, be sure to use plenty of that vegetable, half a pound per person, because vegetables are not very filling.

Implements

Scale to weigh ounces
2-quart glass or ceramic casserole with glass cover
10-inch frying pan or wok
Big, flattened spoon for stirring and serving
Knife for chopping vegetables
Cutting board
1-quart serving bowl

Ingredient	Amount per Person
For Making Rice	
Rice: white or brown	2 ounces
Water	4–5 ounces
For Making Meat	
Canola oil, flour	1 teaspoon each
Knob onions with 6" of stems	$\frac{1}{8}$
Frozen pork tenderloin or boneless chicken breast	1 ounce

For Making Vegetables

Canola oil	1 teaspoon
Mixed vegetables.	12 ounces

Take one from each of the columns below:

Sweet	High-Protein	Veggie	Crunchy
whole baby carrots	peas in pods	broccoli	celery
carrot shreds	green beans	tomatoes	water chestnuts
snap pea pods	lentils*	cauliflower	slivered almonds
asparagus	walnuts	yellow squash	napa cabbage
Alaska peas	frozen tofu	zucchini	bamboo shoots
		greens**	daikon (chinese radish)
		baby corn	bok choi

*Precook. Simmer in plain water for 30 minutes.
**Spinach, chard, kale, escarole, mustard greens, etc.

For Making Sauce

Sour herbal tea (Celestial Seasons Wild Berry Zinger, Red Zinger, or Lemon Zinger, or Bigelow Lemon Lift)	½ cup
Optional, if your stomach tolerates it:	
White vinegar or apple cider vinegar	1–2 tablespoons
Water	½ cup
Honey	1 teaspoon
Cornstarch	1 teaspoon
Bragg Liquid Aminos	2 teaspoons
Low-salt chicken bouillon crystals	½ teaspoon
Can substitute vegetable broth mix powder (Morga or others).	

EARLY PREPARATION

Chop the knob onions or leeks into coins ¼-inch thick, then cut the coins in halves. Put them into a glass jar or plastic container, cover with water, cover with a tightly fitted lid, and store in the refrigerator overnight (can be kept for 3 days). You can substitute Vidalia, walla walla, or Texas Sweet onions for knob onions. These big, sweet varieties of onion are so low in acid that you may be able to digest them without presoaking. On your first try, cut them into large pieces in thin slices so they will contribute flavor to the recipe even if you don't eat the onion itself.

No time to wait overnight for onion purification? Chop the onion finely. Put it in a cup. Douse with a cup of hot water. Let stand 10 minutes. Drain off the strong-smelling liquid, using your finger or a fork to retain the onion. Rinse with a little water, and drain again.

Pick the vegetables you want. There's nothing absolute about the recommendation above to take one from each column. Just take your favorites, keeping in mind that you want a balance of flavors and textures. Not all sweet, not all crunchy—a balance. If you want to save time, pick a prewashed, precut mix like Broccoli Wokly or cruise the salad counter at the supermarket till you have a mix to your heart's content.

IMMEDIATE PREPARATION

Whole vegetables need chopping so they'll cook in short order. Otherwise, you have to perform a mad dervish of sequential cooking like a conductor reaching to cue each player in *Flight of the Bumblebee*. Chop the vegetables to bite-size. For green beans and asparagus, this means pieces no more than an inch long. Plump green beans should be cut half that short, but never cut down the middle or they'll overcook. Don't, however, cut pea pods or else the peas will fall out. Then both the peas and the pods will overcook.

Cauliflower and broccoli you can break by hand into little florets (would that be floret-ettes?) or just chop these cruciferous vegetables about $1/4$-inch thick. Knives work as well as, and maybe faster than, fingers. Don't be intimidated by somebody else's aesthetics about this. Knives don't hurt the taste or nutritional content, and little fans look as pretty as little trees.

COOKING

Make the Wild Berry Zinger tea. Add the honey. Stir it in. Taste it if you want, but don't drink the rest. Put it aside for making the sauce.

To the Chinese, meat means pork unless otherwise specified. This dish is fine with any kind of meat. Start with frozen meat so you can half-thaw it; partially frozen meat cuts more easily. Half-thaw the meat by moving it to the non-freezer part of your refrigerator overnight, or leaving the meat in a metal sink for an hour at room temperature. (If using a microwave, it takes about 4 minutes on Defrost setting per pound of meat). Cut the meat across the grain into slices about an eighth of an inch thick. Cut the slices into bits an eighth of an inch by a half or a whole inch long. This way, you get plenty of flavor out of not much meat, as the Chinese do.

Put the rice and water in the casserole. If you prefer flaky rice, add a teaspoon of oil per person. But remember that this won't hold the sauce well. If it gets sticky anyway, don't get uptight about it. You're not in a Minute Rice ad, and sticky rice is not only okay, it's authentic. A true Chinese cook uses no oil or salt in the rice, and produces rice that sticks to itself so it can be easily eaten with chopsticks—even with sauce in it.

Cover the casserole, heat to boiling, and simmer until all the water is just taken up. White rice takes 15 to 20 minutes, and brown takes 25 to 40. There are many other ways you can cook rice. An electric steamer works well but is a bit slow; use the steamer's directions. If you use a range or microwave, use a casserole that holds at least 3 times as much as your two ingredients so it won't easily boil over. Either way, as soon as the rice water comes to a boil, reduce heat to the lowest possible setting. On the range, this is Warm, not Simmer. In the microwave, this is 1 on a scale of 0 to 10, not Defrost (which is 3 out of 10). A Corning-ware casserole with a glass lid will continue to simmer the rice nicely.

Microwaving cooks rice a little faster than range-top boiling. After white rice comes to a boil, it needs only 13 to 15 minutes of simmering. After brown rice comes to a boil, it needs only about 20 to 30 minutes of simmering.

When the rice has about 10 minutes left to cook, start the skillet or wok (the wok, let's call it) heating on medium-high. Add a teaspoon of oil per person. Drain the onions or leeks so no water can get into the wok and make it spit hot oil into your face. Before the wok gets very hot, add the onions or leeks. Cook 2 to 3 minutes till they start to brown. Immediately add the meat. Spread into a single layer on the wok. Sprinkle flour on top, and salt to taste. When the meat's browning, in half a minute, flip once. After another half a minute, as soon as the meat changes color, remove it from the wok.

Immediately, add the rest of the oil, heat a few seconds, and add all the vegetables. Shake or stir up from the bottom every few seconds for a total of 2 minutes, or until the green vegetables turn dark green. Don't cook longer or they'll lose this color and lose their crunchiness and flavor.

While that 2 minutes of cooking is in progress, stir the cornstarch into the tea (a finger works well; twirling a little wire whisk works too). Add the chicken bouillon crystals and the Bragg Liquid Aminos.

As soon as the veggies turn dark green, add all of the sauce mix, add the onion-fried meat, and stir constantly till it boils. Immediately turn off the heat.

SERVING

Turn out the stir-fry and sauce into a serving bowl. Serve each diner a warm pasta bowl. Part of the charm of eating Chinese style is serving dishes family-style and letting diners serve themselves.

Washing the food down with a dry, astringent tea is the tradition, of course. Serving the same herb tea as used in the stir-fry is also a subtle way of enhancing the flavors.

Light fruit desserts such as sorbet or sliced fruit refresh the palate well. We have found that a salad of fresh fruit served with the Chinese food is even better, refreshing the palate from the strong-tasting hot food throughout the meal. Then the diners need save room in their stomachs only for fortune cookies.

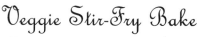

Veggie Stir-Fry Bake

Special thanks to the kitchens of the Parke-Davis Pharmaceutical Research Division of Warner-Lambert Company in Ann Arbor, Michigan, for the inspiration for this recipe. It's one of the few vegetarian main dishes served there. Too satisfying to eat as a side dish, it filled me up on many a Friday's lunch.

Ingredient	Amount to Serve 2
Broccoli	1/4 pound
Pea pods	12
Asparagus	1/4 pound
Portobello mushroom	1 (about 6 ounces)
Green onion	2 small
Fat-free cheddar cheese	4 ounces
Leftover boiled or steamed rice	8 ounces

PREPARATION

One to three days before cooking, chop the green onion into 1/4-inch lengths. Immerse in a cup of water in a glass or plastic bottle, cover tightly, and soak at least overnight. A quick alternative is to chop the onion finely, and soak it in a cup of hot water for 10 minutes.

Prepare (boil or steam) enough rice to leave a cup for leftovers. Use brown rice for a hearty, satisfying taste or, if you want a lighter taste, use white rice. If you want a stronger taste, try Vigo red beans and rice. Just be sure to rinse off the seasonings before cooking, or it may be too spicy for your tummy. The rinsing doesn't have to be thorough; all it takes is putting the rice in the casserole, adding a cup of water, swishing it for a few seconds, and draining off the water while you hold the lid of the casserole on top loosely. Another good alternative for tasty rice is a mix of three parts brown rice and one part wild rice. If you don't have any preprepared, put $1/3$ cup of Uncle Ben's Converted brown rice and $2/3$ cup of water in a small glass or ceramic casserole, put it in a microwave, heat to boiling (use High for 3 minutes), and boil for 20 minutes per package directions.

COOKING

Start about 20 minutes before you want to eat lunch or dinner. Drain the water off the chopped onion. In a wok or 10-inch skillet, put a teaspoons of canola oil and 2 ounces of water and heat on Medium High till the water starts to boil. Add the onion and boil, uncovered, until the water has boiled away and the onion is lightly browned.

While the onion boils, chop the other vegetables. Cut the broccoli into pieces no more than an inch long and with pieces of stems $1/4$-inch thick. Cut the pea pods into quarters. Cut the asparagus into pieces $1/2$-inch long. Cut the stem off the portobello mushroom, and chop it into 1-inch by $1/2$-inch by $1/2$-inch hunks.

Add a tablespoon of canola oil to the wok as soon as the onion is lightly browned, and add all the vegetables. Stir and fry for a minute until the color of the green vegetables deepens.

Take a cup of hot cooked (steamed or boiled) rice. Put the rice in a range-safe ceramic casserole. Add a tablespoon of Bragg Liquid Aminos, $1/4$ teaspoon NuSalt, and a dash of black pepper. Stir for a few seconds. Add all the vegetables. Toss to mix well. Grate 4 ounces of fat-free cheddar and spread it over the top.

Heat on the range a minute or two until you hear a few sounds of boiling (or microwave uncovered on High for 2 minutes). Bake in a preheated oven at 425° for 8 minutes or until the cheese starts to brown. Let the dish cool for 5 minutes before you try to eat it.

SERVING

This recipe makes 24 ounces, a pint and a half. It should be enough to feed two people as a main dish or four as a side dish. When I first made it, no one was home but me, and I couldn't resist finishing the whole thing. If you want it to go farther, you can double the amounts of rice, Braggs, Nu Salt, and cheese. This is more like the institutional version that I first tasted and tried to improve. But why skimp on the vegetables?

Chicken Portobello Belle

No, this isn't named after the Mark Knopfler tune. It's named after the por-tobello mushrooms that cover the chicken and after Belle, who encouraged me to try this recipe when I couldn't find a recipe for Chicken Cordon Bleu.

Ingredient	Amount to Serve 2
Wild rice	1 ounce
Brown rice	3 ounces
Hot water	8 ounces
Chicken bouillon powder	1 teaspoon
Dried chopped chives	1 tablespoon
Turkey Canadian bacon	1 ounce, in medium-thin slices
Fat-free Swiss cheese slices	3 ounces
Chicken breast halves	2, about $2/3$–$3/4$ pound
Portobello mushroom	1, sliced about $1/8$-inch thick
Cracker crumbs	2 tablespoons
Salt or NuSalt	$1/4$ teaspoon
Ground black pepper	$1/8$ teaspoon
Cream sherry	4 tablespoons
NuSalt	
Freshly ground black or mixed peppercorns	
Buttery-flavor cooking spray	

PREPARATION AND COOKING

Put the rices into a shallow, range-safe ceramic casserole. Add the hot water and the chicken bouillon powder. Stir a little. Put on a glass lid so you can watch. Heat on the range at medium-high (in microwave on High) until it starts to boil (about 2 minutes). Reduce heat to simmer. ('Waving: Stop it and reset the heat setting to Low; 2 out of 10 is enough.) Simmer for 20 minutes.

While you wait for the rice, pound the chicken breast halves out with a hammer so they'll cover most of the inside of the casserole. Cut most of the stem off the Portabello mushroom, and slice the mushroom fairly thinly.

When the rice has simmered for 20 minutes, not all the water will be taken up, but most of it should be, and the rice should look pretty plump. While it's hot, spread the following on top of the rice in the order given: the chives, the turkey Canadian bacon, the Swiss cheese slices, the chicken breast halves, NuSalt and pepper to taste, the mushroom slices, and the cracker crumbs. Put a tablespoon of cream sherry down each corner of the casserole. Spray the cracker crumbs with the cook-ing spray till they look yellow, maybe 15 seconds.

Cover the casserole again, and heat on the range at medium-high (or microwave on High) for 5 minutes. Stock in the bottom of the casserole should be visibly boiling. Move it to a 400° oven and heat it there for 10 minutes. Remove the lid. Broil for 3 to 5 minutes until the outer edges of the mushroom darken well but don't burn.

SERVING

Slide a big spatula under the chicken and rice. Remove a serving. Slide it right side up onto a plate. Accompany with fruit salad.

Jim's Rice Stuffing

My son Jim likes wild rice a lot, so he created a stuffing that sticks together like a bread stuffing, but has hardly any bread in it. It's so nutritious that it can be served as a main dish, but it's even better cooked as a real stuffing— steamed and moistened inside a roasting turkey or chicken.

Ingredient	Amount to Serve 4
Brown rice	4 ounces
Wild rice	1 ounce
Hot water	12 ounces
Baby carrots	4
Crimini or button mushrooms	6 medium
Celery	1 large stalk or 2 small
Vegit®*	2 shakes
Salt or NuSalt	pinch
White or wheat bread, dry	2 ounces
or Fat-free saltines	12

PREPARATION AND COOKING

Put the two rices and the water in a small, deep, glass or ceramic casserole. Cover well with a glass cover (or a pierced piece of plastic wrap in the microwave). Heat to boiling at a range setting of medium-high (or in a microwave). Simmer (if microwaving, at very low setting, 2 out of a maximum of 10). If you use Uncle Ben's parboiled brown rice, 20 minutes is enough. Otherwise, simmer for 30 to 35 minutes. In either case, cook until the water is almost all absorbed by the rice.

While the rices are cooking, prepare the vegetables. Grate the carrots or chop them into bits no thicker than a paper match. Wash the mushrooms and trim off the tough ends of their stems. Slice the trimmed mushrooms about $1/8$-inch thick. Chop the celery into little bits about the size of a baby pea (a square pea).

Break the walnuts by hand into 4 to 6 bits per nutmeat, big enough to chew.

Coarsely grate the very dry white or wheat bread or (easier) crush the fat-free saltines by hand. (Crush them in a plastic bag, or right in the sleeve in which they're packaged.)

Pull the rice off the heat (or out of the microwave) as soon as it's done enough. Take off the lid. Add the vegetables and walnuts, and mix briefly with a fork. Add the bread (or cracker) crumbs and 2 ounces of hot water. Mix very little, just enough to get the crumbs into the stuffing.

For stuffing cooked by itself, cover the stuffing with the lid again. This is not a stuffing that browns, so don't leave it uncovered. That would make some of the rice tough enough to be dangerous to your dental fillings. Bake at 400° for 30 minutes.

For stuffing a fowl, first reheat the stuffing. Toss on medium-high heat till it just begins to fizzle (a minute or two). Or, if microwaving, cover it and heat on High for a minute or so until it's almost too hot to touch. Spoon heated stuffing while still hot into the bird's body cavity. The hot stuffing helps the bird to cook in the most sanitary way.

For cooking the stuffing with No-Name Chicken, see that recipe (in Chapter 21).

*Caution: Vegit® contains some stomach offenders.

Chapter 21

ℱAMILY
FAVORITE DINNERS

This chapter starts with finger-food appetizers and some of our family's most-requested meat and fish recipes. Then follows a veg-by-veg account of how to cook the common vegetables simply, quickly, and preserving their nutritional value while making them exceptionally digestible. Recipes are followed by suggestions on how to sauce, spice, and serve them.

APPETIZERS

Most appetizers are grossly fatty batter-dipped and fried concoctions. They stave off hunger because of their fat content and because of their protein content—the chicken, shrimp, cheese, or whatever beneath the breading. This isn't to recommend fatty appetizers, but there are some delicious ways to get enough easy-to-eat protein to help keep the guests out of the kitchen until dinner is ready.

Before dinner, or instead of a lunch entree, we sometimes have one of the following appetizers. Crackers, especially fat-free ones such as SnackWell's Pepper Crackers or Wheat Crackers, make the dipping more fun and the chewing more satisfying than bread.

Salmon Dip

See Chapter 19, Potatoes and Potato-Based Dishes, for this recipe. It can also be made with canned or freshly cooked tuna. Swordfish is okay, too, as long as it is chopped finely. All these fishes taste strong enough to stand up to the yogurt in the dip. Be sure to taste it before you set it out for others. If it's too fishy for you, double the amount of yogurt in the mix, or add as much fat-free cream cheese.

─────────── ✲✲ ───────────

Low-Fat Chicken Liver Pate

Surprise—the elegance of a homemade pate is available without most of the fat and cholesterol! The pretty mauve color, the light but firm texture, the exotic taste, even the groovy pattern that forms on it as it bakes are all inviting. Just keep your portion size down—share it with a couple of friends—and it won't put the bad stuff on your coronaries.

Ingredient	Amount
Liver from 3–4-pound chicken	1
Egg substitute	3 ounces (equivalent to 1 1/2 eggs)
Breadspread	2 ounces
Port or red wine	1 tablespoon
Ground nutmeg	pinch
Ground ginger	pinch
Salt or NuSalt	1/4 teaspoon
Freshly ground pepper	pinch

Preheat oven to 300°. Blend all ingredients well in a small electric blender. Beat on medium-high for half a minute or until moderately foamy. With aluminum foil, tightly wrap the outside (down-side) of one Texas-size muffin holder and mold the extra to form a flat spill-catching lip. Carefully pull the foil off the muffin-holder and tuck it into one of the two middle muffin-holders of six in the Texas muffin pan. Fill the foil pan liner with the pate mix. Bake for 40 to 50 minutes or until the center has risen and won't quiver when the pan is jiggled slightly. Cool, invert onto a saucer, peel away the foil, and serve.

─────────── ✲✲ ───────────

Catfish Fingers

This makes a good TV-watching snack. Buy fresh catfish nuggets at your fish market. Expect 4 to 6 servings per pound if you're using this as an appetizer.

Ingredient	Amount to Serve 2
Catfish nuggets	½ pound
Flour	2 tablespoons
Kraft Free grated topping or other fat-free, finely grated parmesan	2 tablespoons
Freshly ground pepper	¼ teaspoon

Wash the catfish nuggets in cold water. Drain but don't completely dry them on paper towels. Put the flour, grated parmesan, and pepper into a bag. Grab the bag by its neck to keep it shut. Shake a dozen times. Reopen the bag. Add two or three catfish nuggets at a time, close the bag loosely again, and shake to coat the nuggets.

Heat a 10-inch nonstick skillet on medium heat. Spray it lightly with Pam or other vegetable oil spray if desired. Don't worry about the breaded catfish sticking; enough fat cooks out of them to "fry" them. When the skillet is up to temperature, arrange all the coated catfish nuggets over its surface. Cook for 2 to 4 minutes, until the down-side is a golden brown. Flip the nuggets and cook the other side for a little less time, till it's golden also.

After the fish fingers are cooked, sprinkle with salt or NuSalt to taste. Serve with Honey Mustard Yogurt Dressing or Ranch Dressing (see Chapter 16, Salad Specials). Garnish with Louise's Fat-Free Potato Chips or, for a heartier treat, with French "Fries" (see Chapter 19, Potatoes and Potato-Based Dishes).

Chicken Fingers

Ingredient	Amount to Serve 2
Boneless, skinless chicken breast	1
Flour	¼ cup
Kraft Free grated topping or other fat-free, finely grated parmesan	¼ cup
(Can substitute cracker crumb or crushed corn flakes, if desired.)	
Freshly ground pepper	¼ teaspoon
Plain yogurt	4 ounces
Ground rosemary and thyme	¼ teaspoon each

Heat a toaster oven or broiler to 450°.

Wash the the chicken breast in cold water. Dry on paper towels. Cut chicken into ¼-inch slices.

Put yogurt and ground herbs into a shallow bowl. Mix them with a fork. With the same fork, dredge the chicken slices through the yogurt mix. Put the flour, grated parmesan, and pepper in a small bowl. Stir with a fork. Dredge the chicken through this coating, one slice at a time. Arrange all the coated and dipped chicken slices in a broiling pan, so the top surface of the chicken is 1 to 2 inches away from the heating element. Broil for 3 to 5 minutes until the top side is a golden brown. Flip the chicken slices and broil the other side for a little less time, till it's golden also.

After the chicken is cooked, sprinkle with salt or NuSalt to taste. Serve with Honey Mustard Yogurt Dressing or Ranch Dressing (see Chapter 16, Salad Specials). Garnish with Louise's Fat-Free Potato Chips. For a heartier treat or for lunch, serve with French "Fries" (see Chapter 19, Potatoes and Potato-Based Dishes).

𝒟INNER ENTREES

𝒩o-𝒩ame Chicken or 𝒩o-𝒩ame Turkey

Our family never came up with a name for this way of cooking a chicken. The chicken is sort of roasted from on top, sort of steamed from underneath, and sort of fried, so naming it by cooking method wouldn't be easy. "No-Name Chicken" identifies it enough for us. We used to make it with cut-up fryers with the skin on, in a big 10-inch skillet that could go in the oven. You'll find that the skinless all-white-meat version here is surprisingly juicy.

Ingredient	Amount to Serve 2
Chicken breast halves or turkey breast	2, about ⅔–¾ pound
Flour	2 tablespoons
Salt or NuSalt	¼ teaspoon
Ground black pepper	⅛ teaspoon
Breadspread	2 tablespoons

Tools

Small glass or ceramic casserole dish

Kitchen mallet, meat tenderizing hammer, or other pounder

PREPARATION

Make Jim's Rice Stuffing (Chapter 20). If you are pressed for time or want a plainer dish, make Simple Bread Stuffing (Chapter 17) instead. Pound the chicken breasts until they are about half as thick as they were. Be careful to keep the thickness of the meat as even as possible. Pound the same way if you are using half a turkey breast. Ready-to-grill turkey breast slices need not be pounded.

Separately, mix the flour, salt or NuSalt, and black pepper.

Leave the stuffing in the same little casserole in which it was mixed for final cooking. Cover the stuffing, which should be hot already, with the meat. Cover the stuffing entirely so it doesn't dry out. The meat can overlap a bit, because it shrinks as it cooks. Cover the meat (and any uncovered stuffing) by sprinkling the flour, salt, and pepper mixture over it. Even out the coverage with a fork or spoon.

COOKING

Place the dish in a 425° oven. After 5 minutes, pull the dish out part way and spread the breadspead all over the flour mixture, till it is all "wetted."

Don't want to spread stuff around in a hot dish in a hot oven? Okay, skip the step above. Before starting to cook, spray the flour mixture with buttery-flavor cooking spray until it is well covered (about 10 seconds).

Bake at 425° for 35 to 40 minutes or until no pink shows when the meat is stabbed in the middle with a sharp knife.

SERVING

Serve with baked (or microwaved) sweet potatoes and a green vegetable. I like having a plainer carbo with dinners too; so I sometimes serve this with baked potatoes or fresh bread.

Ron's Chicken Vesuvio

My older brother sent me his version of this tasty Italian recipe. Toned down for my own stomach, it's still piquant and interesting.

Ingredient	Amount to Serve 4
Boneless, skinless chicken breast halves (Amish)	4
Finely chopped onion	¼ cup

Baking potatoes	3 large or 4 medium, sliced into 6–8 chunks each
Coating Mix	
Flour	$\frac{1}{3}$ cup
Ground basil	1 $\frac{1}{2}$ teaspoons
Ground oregano	1 teaspoon
Vegit®*	dash
Thyme	$\frac{1}{4}$ teaspoon
Pepper	$\frac{1}{4}$ teaspoon
Paprika	dash
Sage	pinch
Rosemary	pinch
Chicken bouillon crystals	1 teaspoon
Hot water	1 cup
Dry white wine	$\frac{3}{8}$ cup

Preheat oven to 425°. Presoak chopped onion in 1 cup of hot water for at least 10 minutes. Drain. Pat dry. Combine dry ingredients in a large, shallow pan. Add onion.

Wash chicken and pat dry. Coat chicken lightly with coating mix and onions. Spray with buttery-flavor cooking spray. Put chicken into a large, shallow baking pan. Place potatoes among and around the chicken. Bake for 20 minutes or until chicken browns slightly.

Add 1 cup of water and bouillon crystals to leftover coating mix. Whisk to blend. Pour into skillet. Add wine. Heat at medium, stirring constantly, until it thickens. Ladle over chicken and potatoes. Sprinkle with parsley and $\frac{1}{4}$ cup grated parmesan cheese. Reduce oven temperature to 375°. Bake for another 20 minutes or until potatoes and chicken are fork-tender.

Serve with pan juices.

*Caution: Vegit® contains some stomach offenders.

Broiled Salmon with Herbs

Ingredient	Amount per Person
Salmon	$\frac{1}{4}$–$\frac{1}{3}$ pound
Plain nonfat yogurt	$\frac{1}{2}$ cup
Savory or tarragon	$\frac{1}{2}$–1 teaspoon

Other Herbs to Try:

Chives (dried)

Dill (dry or fresh)

Herbs fines (French herb mix)

Salmon has a stronger taste than most fish and can be terribly dry, especially Pacific salmon. Cooking and serving with a sauce helps make salmon delicious. Here's a basic recipe and some variations to try.

PURCHASE

Pick either fillets (boneless but with skin) or steaks (with bones, including part of the spine, and skin) at a grocery store you trust. Choose whatever is in season—chum (beige, cheapest, least flavor), king (orange, expensive, most flavor), Chinook, etc. It can vary from a light beige to a bright salmon orange without having anything wrong with it. Just make sure as you look at the fish that the color is even and there are no semitransparent spots. When you receive it from the counterperson, don't be shy: Smell it to make sure it has no strong smell. Flash-frozen can be as good as "fresh," which is often really thawed, previously frozen salmon. Get ¼ to ⅜ of a pound (including skin and bone) per person, not more, because salmon is fatty as fish goes and it's very filling.

STORAGE

Store unfrozen salmon in the refrigerator in a plastic bag covered with ice cubes in a deep pan. A covered loaf pan works best. This keeps it around 32° instead of refrigerator temperature, which may be as high as 40°. Keep for not for more than 24 hours. Otherwise, it starts to get that fishy smell and taste characteristic of compounds called amines. Amine smells mean that the fish is deteriorating and you shouldn't eat it.

PREPARATION

Take the grilling rack and the drip-catching pan out of your toaster oven. Preheat on the Broil setting for 3 to 5 minutes while you do the cooking preparations that follow. Pour just enough warm water into the drip-catching pan to cover the bottom, about ⅓ cup. Put the toaster oven's slotted sheet metal (or wire) grilling rack on the pan.

Wash the surface of the salmon. Running water is enough. To wash steaks, use a brush or sponge, not your fingers, because steaks have sharp, transparent bones that stick out obliquely and can poke you. Put the slices of salmon, separated an inch from one another, on the slotted grilling rack.

Make the sauce, ½ cup per serving. Mix the yogurt and herbs with a slotted spoon, just enough to disperse the herbs well. Put half of the sauce into a serving bowl.

Cover the top surface of the salmon slices generously with sauce; spread it as thick as apple butter, but not as thick as frosting. The surface should look white, not pink.

COOKING

Slide the pan of sauced salmon gently into the toaster oven so the water in the pan doesn't spill. Broil 15 to 25 minutes, until three things happen: 1) The edges of the sauce get browned a little. 2) The salmon changes to a light-orange cooked color uniformly (including the bottom). 3) The salmon flakes easily. Slide a table knife under the middle of a slice of salmon and lift a little, slowly and gently. The salmon slice should start to break, not raise stiffly. A fork stuck in the middle and twisted makes the salmon open up and flake. A knife inserted into the middle of the salmon goes through cleanly and easily.

SERVING

While the salmon is broiling on top and grilling and steaming from beneath, set an oven to 150° and put serving plates in it (separated, not stacked) to warm. As soon as the salmon passes the three tests above, serve it immediately on a warmed plate. Put a ¼-cup dollop of sauce next to it in a little bowl for dipping, or just serve the bowl of sauce with it.

ACCOMPANIMENTS

This salmon dish goes well with panned spinach, steamed asparagus, or stir-fried Broccoli Wokly. For starches, try baked potatoes with nonfat sour cream and the same herbs as used on the salmon, or Rice Erroneous.

Hunter's Chicken

My kids asked for this all-in-one-pot dish on many a Sunday. They'd give me grief if it were not included in a book of family faves, so here goes. The Rombauer-Becker version is also called chicken cacciatore or chicken chasseur.

Ingredient	Amount to Serve 2
Chopped onion, presoaked	¼ cup
Skinless Amish chicken breasts	2
Salt or NuSalt	¼ teaspoon

Black or white pepper	⅛ teaspoon
Canola oil	1 teaspoon
Tomato wedges	1 pound
Fresh celery	½ stalk
Carrot	2 small or 1 large
Bay leaf	½ leaf
Thyme	⅛ teaspoon
Marjoram	⅛ teaspoon
Mushrooms	4 ounces
Chicken bouillon crystals	1 teaspoon
Water	1 cup
Sweet white wine	2 tablespoons
Flour	1 tablespoon

PREPARATION AND COOKING

Presoak chopped onion (Texas Sweet, Vidalia, or green) in 1 cup of hot water per ¼ cup of onion, for 20 minutes. Pour off the water. Put the oil in a soup pot. Add the drained onions. Sauté on Medium until lightly browned. Remove from pot.

Wash chicken and pat dry. Put in soup pot. Cover. Heat at Medium-high until browned well on both sides. Add tomato, carrot, celery, chicken bouillon crystals, water, wine, herbs, and browned onions. Bring to a boil and reduce heat to low. Simmer 20 to 30 minutes or until chicken is tender.

SERVING

Serve with spaghetti or white rice, a green salad with Italian dressing or red wine vinegar and olive oil, and crusty bread. White grape juice is good with this.

Chicken Paprikas

Pop'-ri-kosh is the way to say this Hungarian dish. This version is authentic except for all the saturated fat associated with the original. It's very digestible and tasty. With the sauce, you won't miss the skin on the chicken.

Ingredient	Amount to Serve 2
Chopped onion, presoaked	¼ cup
Skinless Amish chicken breasts	2
Salt or NuSalt	¼ teaspoon

Black or white pepper	⅛ teaspoon
Canola oil	1 teaspoon
Sweet Hungarian paprika	1 teaspoon
Mushrooms	4 ounces
Chicken bouillon crystals	1 teaspoon
Water	1 cup
Dry white wine	½ cup
Flour	1 tablespoon
Nonfat sour cream	½ cup

PREPARATION AND COOKING

Presoak chopped onion (Texas Sweet, Vidalia, or green) in 1 cup of hot water per ¼ cup of onion, for at least 10 minutes. Pour off the water. Put the oil in a skillet big enough to hold all the chicken pieces. Add the drained onions. Sauté on Medium until lightly browned. Remove from pan. Add mushrooms to skillet. Cook on Medium heat until tender, about 1 to 2 minutes. Remove from pan. Wash chicken and pat dry. Combine flour and spices in paper bag. Add chicken pieces and shake to coat. Spray moderately with buttery cooking spray. Put in skillet. Cover. Heat at Medium-High until browned well on both sides. Add chicken bouillon crystals, water, and wine. Add paprika and onions last. Stir. Bring to a boil and reduce heat to low. Simmer 20 to 30 minutes or until chicken is tender. Remove chicken from pan. Stir flour with nonfat sour cream. Stir mixture into pan juices. Heat very slowly until thickened. Do not heat to boiling or the sour cream will become runny and thready. Pour sauce over chicken.

SERVING

Serve with noodles, a green vegetable, and crusty bread. A strong-tasting, dark red grape juice is good with this.

Mahimahi with Coriander Butter Sauce

Ingredient	Amount per Person
Mahimahi	¼–⅓ pound
Breadspread	½ cup
Ground coriander	¼–½ teaspoon

PREPARATION AND COOKING

Mahimahi is a rich, white fish. Fillets of it come fairly thick, ready to broil. It is a firm-textured fish that breaks into big flakes like salmon when cooked. Unlike salmon, it is delicate-tasting, so adding a fairly strong taste to it can complement it. The simple coriander sauce used in this recipe tastes very much like lemon pepper, but it's not apt to upset the stomach.

PURCHASE, STORAGE, PREPARATION

Buy, store, and prepare mahimahi for broiling in a toaster oven as for salmon, except to make a different sauce.

CORIANDER BUTTER SAUCE

In a small bowl, mix the breadspread and coriander with a fork. Remove half. Spread half of this half on top of the fish before broiling.

COOKING

Start broiling as for salmon, but expect this fish, which comes in smaller, somewhat thinner pieces than salmon, to cook faster. After 6 minutes of broiling, pull the cooking tray part way out of the toaster oven. With a spatula as big as the fillets, turn them over. Cover the top surface with the rest of the coriander butter sauce. Broil for another 6 to 8 minutes or until the fish passes three tests: 1) The edges of the fillet get browned a little. 2) The mahimahi uniformly changes color slightly to an opaque whiter color. 3) The mahimahi flakes easily. Slide a table knife under the middle of a fillet and lift a little, slowly. The fillet should start to break, not raise stiffly. A fork stuck in the middle and twisted makes the fish open up and flake. Work gently or the fillet will break into pieces.

SERVING

Heat the unused remainder of the coriander butter sauce until it melts and pour it into little cups to pour on the mahimahi. Serve the fish with the sauce on plates heated in a 150° oven.

ACCOMPANIMENTS

Steam or microwave a sweet, delicate vegetable such as baby carrots or snow peas in pods. A delicate starch is good, too. Try boiled or steamed brown rice, or boil 2 ounces of orzo (rice-shaped pasta) and serve mixed with a teaspoon of canola oil per person.

Cooking Vegetables

The following general directions are for using my three favorite ways of cooking vegetables. They are steaming, stir-frying, and (if you fear not the smattering of adverse nutritional reports) microwaving. We'll also get into specifics for each of the commonly cooked vegetables.

Steaming

On the Range

Steaming is a great way to cook vegetables quickly, preserving their nutritional value and taste. You can do it easily on the range.

Rangetop Method. All you need is a steamer rack and a 1- or 2-quart saucepan with a tight lid. Put the steamer rack in the saucepan. Add ¼ inch of hot water—not enough to leave any water in contact with the steamer rack. Put washed vegetables into the rack. Heat the water to boiling, then turn the heat down to low (enough to keep steam rising). Carefully, to avoid getting burned by live steam, sample the vegetables periodically. As soon as the vegetables are tender-crisp, remove the saucepan from heat, leave the cover off, and cool the vegetables on the rack in the saucepan with some cool running water so they don't overcook.

Cooking Time. The smaller the vegetable pieces, the more quickly and evenly they cook. You can serve large vegetables whole if you want to; it just takes longer to steam them.

Electric Steamer Method. These new appliances are very handy. They perform consistently, and cleanup is easy. A coworker of mine once gifted us with what he called an "electric brick." It appeared to be an ordinary brick except for having an electric cord attached. It was inscribed, "This is an electric brick. It will do anything that an ordinary brick does, but it does it *electrically.*"

This is very similar in principle to the electric vegetable steamer. It does anything that an ordinary steamer does, but it does so electrically. There are two important things to know about electric steamers: First, steam for less time than the directions say. Try half to three-quarters of the recommended time. Go longer only after you sample the results. Sample carefully with a fork or tongs so you don't get burned by live steam.

The second piece of hard-earned advice about electric steamers is that you need to rinse the whole thing out and wash it after each use. Water condenses down in a drip-catcher during steaming. It carries enough of the nutrients from the vegetables that it smells terrible after a couple of days if you don't wash it.

Cooking Time. The recipes that follow give cooking times for microwaving vegetables. They are also applicable to the steamer, because in effect the microwave is used as a steamer.

STIR-FRYING

All vegetables that can be cut small can be stir-fried. Cut non-leafy vegetables into pieces no more than an inch long and a quarter of an inch in diameter. The following groups of vegetables each take about the same length of time to stir-fry:

One minute or less. Mushrooms, mung bean sprouts, peas, tomato wedges, zucchini, squash, kale, spinach, other dark green, leafy vegetables.

Two to three minutes. Asparagus, green beans, broccoli, cauliflower, celery, Swiss chard, bok choi, pea pods.

Three to five minutes. Baby carrots, daikon, similar-sized pieces of the vegetables just above.

The pros recommend using a tablespoon of oil per serving. Heat it in a skillet or wok on medium-high until it rolls around looking watery-thin instead of thick and oily. Add the vegetables in one big dump, all at once and right in the middle of the pot, so any water with them does not make the pot spit hot oil at you. Flip the vegetables over every 15 to 30 seconds, or shake the pot so that the vegetables turn over.

If vegetables are insufficiently cooked for your taste after the times given above, add ¼ cup of hot water per serving, cover, bring to a boil, reduce heat to low, and let steam for a minute or two.

MICROWAVING WITHOUT BURNING

As a way of cooking vegetables, the microwave has been hissed and dissed by cooks and nutritionists alike. It burns the tips of the veggies. It kills the vitamins. Maybe it even makes carcinogens and twists fatty acids and amino acids into bad forms. Well, sure, cook vegetables by following the directions that come with the microwave and it does a horrible job. But don't blame the microwave for all of that. Blame in part the cooks who write the books. All they seem to do is to blast the vegetables and keep them dry. This may preserve the vegetables from the growth of any form of life, but so would nuclear fission. Maybe this version of microwaving is why people refer to microwaving as "nuking."

General Method. We're going to do two things differently. First, instead of cooking vegetables without water or with only the water that clings to them when washed, we're going to add a little water before cooking. A tablespoon per serving is enough. This helps steam the vegetables and keep them from superheating (scorching). Second, we're going to blast the vegetables only to the boiling point; then we're going to dial down.

First, do a pilot study. Put an 8-ounce cup of cold water in a clear glass cup—a Pyrex measuring cup, for instance. Set it uncovered in the middle of your microwave. Set the oven for 3 minutes on High. Start the oven and watch progress through the window. Note the exact time when the water starts boiling. Three minutes minus this time is your heating time for 'waving most of the vegetables in the following recipes. We're going to pretend that vegetables are all water (which is very close to the truth; they're mostly water). We're going to heat veggies to boiling on High, then we're not going to blast them further. We're going to *simmer* them till almost cooked. Then we'll let the steam that remains finish the job.

BROCCOLI, CAULIFLOWER, OR BROCCOFLOWER

Wash in cool water. Break florets into small pieces. The heads should be no bigger than the end of your thumb. The stalk should be no longer than an inch, and no thicker than a pen. Main stalks are yummy too. Cut off their tough hide one side at a time with a big knife, or peel it back from the end. Then chop the pieces into quarters lengthwise, one to three inches long and no more than ½-inch thick.

Weigh the broccoli on a scale that reads in ounces. Put the broccoli into a ceramic bowl just big enough to hold it—a Corningware GrabIt is fine, or another small bowl. Add a tablespoon of water. Cover loosely. A Corelle saucer or dessert plate works fine. Keep the "lid" right side up if you can; it'll stay on better and it will drip condensate back into the bowl instead of out the edges. Heat in the microwave on High according to the following formula: [Time to heat 8 ounces of water to boiling] X [Number of ounces of broccoli/8].

Okay, okay, you don't want to follow a formula. Then cook 8 ounces of broccoli and heat it on High for the length of time it took to boil your cup of water. If you're cooking more broccoli, add a minute for every 4 ounces extra.

Next, immediately heat the broccoli on the $^3/_{10}$ (defrost) setting for another 2 to 3 minutes: 2 minutes if you like your broccoli a little crunchy, 3 if you like it tender. Leave the oven off **and** the vegetables covered for at least 3 minutes. Serve with breadspread, nonfat sour cream, plain yogurt, or low-fat cheese sauce.

ASPARAGUS

You can despair of getting asparagus to cook decently. The tips are mushy or the stalks are tough, or both. Rombauer and Becker had me tying bunches together so they'd stand upright, then steaming them in a tall container. This is impossible or exotic beyond an ordinary person's means, unless you happen to have a coffee pot that doesn't smell like coffee and you like a lot of trouble.

The microwave can make it easy. Store asparagus upright in a glass of water in the fridge, the tops covered loosely with plastic. It's good for a couple of days this way, but gets dry on top and mushy on the bottom in a week. Wash off any sand that adheres in the tips. Snap off the tough ends by hand. Prepare half a pound this way.

Throwing gourmet-dom to the winds, break the stalks in half. Put the thick-ended pieces in a Corningware or other ceramic bowl just big enough to hold them and the tops. Add a tablespoon of cool water. Cover loosely, with a glass lid, a Corelle saucer, or other small dish that is microwave-safe. Microwave on High for 2 minutes. Let stand a minute until the live steam dissipates. With tools and an oven mitt, remove the lid. Toss the asparagus tips on top. Microwave on High for another 2 minutes. Let stand for no more than a minute before you uncover carefully with mitt and tools. Serve plain or with nonfat sour cream. Don't fight with your spouse for all the tips.

GREEN BEANS

Tough, sullen little villains when microwaved dry, green beans can be sweet and tender, just like Mama used to make, if you are willing to add enough water. Green beans should be broken into pieces no more than an inch long so they cook evenly. Put them in a bowl that is at least 3 times as wide as it is high. Add enough water so that the beans are *almost* covered, *almost* floating. Add a loose lid. Heat to boiling on High, keeping in mind how much water there is. (If you use 8 ounces of green beans, you'll need another 8 ounces of water, so you have to heat for about 5 minutes on High to make it boil). Simmer for another 7 to 10 minutes, depending on how thick the beans are. Serve with the liquid and melt 1 to 2 teaspoons of breadspread in it. Encourage the diners to get the best flavor and vitamins from the beans by serving the beans in bowls with spoons, instead of on plates, to be eaten with forks.

BUTTERNUT SQUASH, YAMS, AND SWEET POTATOES

These are the vegetables to cook on High in the microwave. Ounce for ounce, they all take about the same amount of cooking.

Butternut Squash. The squash should be cut in half with a big, sharp knife. With a large steel spoon, scoop out the seeds. Lay each half with the open face down on a Corningware or other microwave-safe plate. 'Wave on High for 4 minutes. Rotate the plate a quarter-turn in the oven and wave for another 4 minutes or until the inside is as soft as you like. Let it cool for a few minutes till you can handle it, or put on a potholder mitt. Scoop out the cooked squash from the tough, dark green rind. In a bowl, mash the cooked squash with 2 tablespoons of breadspread. Return the squash to the rind. Sprinkle with cinnamon and brown sugar or honey if desired. Serve.

Yams and Sweet Potatoes. These should be cleaned lightly with a scrub brush. Cut out bigger discolored areas, if any, so their off-taste does not affect the overall taste. Pierce small tubers once, big ones in three places. Set on a saucer in the microwave. If you are cooking three or more tubers at a time, arrange them in a circle, end to end. 'Wave on High for 2 minutes for one medium-sized tuber, 3 minutes for two medium or one large, 4 minutes for three medium tubers, or 5 minutes for four medium or two large. Flip them over. Repeat 'waving. When they stop steamin' and screamin', tap with the bottom of a tablespoon or push on them quickly with your finger. They're done when they are soft. Served plain, they may be sweet enough for you. Adding a dab of breadspread and a few crumbled pecans makes them special.

PANNED KALE, SPINACH, CHARD, BEET TOPS, AND OTHER GREENS

Nutritionists worship the dark green, leafy vegetables because of their vitamins, minerals, and other heroic organic cofactors. A basic problem, however, is how to prepare them so they are not tough, not limp, and not hard to digest. The secret is to cook them just a little and not to lose the good nutrition in the cooking water.

Take about 4 ounces of fresh greens per serving. Wash well in running water. Shake off the excess but do not blot or spin dry. In a large skillet, put 1 teaspoon of olive oil. Add your favorite heavy-duty seasoning to cope with the strongish flavor of the greens. Suggested additions: 1 teaspoon of onion, presoaked in hot water for 10 minutes and drained; ½ teaspoon Vegit®*; or ½ teaspoon mixed oregano and thyme per serving. When the oil is hot, add the greens and cover immediately. Shake and cook on Medium-High for half a minute to a minute after it comes back to a boil (steam rises). Immediately turn out into a serving bowl.

This quick method of cooking in a pan is sometimes called *panning*.

*Caution: Vegit® contains some stomach offenders.

Chapter 22

𝒟ESSERTS
YOU DESERVE

𝒯he trouble with most desserts is that they can make you pay too high a price for a few minutes of enjoyment. If they're high in fat, as most cooked desserts are, you pay the price in unwanted additions to your waist, thighs, and coronaries. If they're high in sugar, they raise your blood sugar too far and this makes your pancreas dump a ton of insulin into your bloodstream to cope with the overload of sugar. Then, an hour or two after you eat, the insulin has made your fat cells drink up all the glucose and change it into more—yes, you guessed, it—**fat**. You ate lots of sugar, you thought it would give you energy, and instead you just gain weight and—yes, *feel hungry again*. The insulin does such a good job that your bloodstream gets deprived once again of glucose, and you feel crabby, weak, and hungry. Do that often enough and you get fat. Or worse, you can develop diabetes.

How can you enjoy desserts and not get this reaction, this cascade of events with unpleasant consequences? There are a couple of secrets. Sucrose, ordinary table sugar, is the serious culprit. It has no off-tastes, it's just a pure chemical. Great for flavoring things if you just want them sweeter, except for two things. One is that it's not very sweet, compared with a few other sugars. That means you have to take in more calories of it to get the taste you want. The other is that, the more of it that you eat, the less you notice how sweet it is, and therefore, the more of it you eat. Try doing without sugar for a week. Then have a soda. I swear, you'll gag at how sweet it is. Ordinarily you don't notice the sweetness,because your taste buds become tolerant of the taste.

A sweeter sugar is fructose, fruit sugar. It somehow forestalls hunger (see Chapter 7 for details). Don't get hooked on it and use tablespoons of it a day; some sketchy evidence suggests that it could be hard on the liver.

Another idea is to have your sugar flavored. Use brown sugar, turbinado sugar, honey, or thawed frozen apple juice concentrate. Dr. Dean Ornish says you're likely to get sick of the taste of these before you eat so much that it harms you.

Finally, if all else fails and you want plain, unadulterated sugar, try using powdered sugar instead of granulated sugar. It's fluffed up half again as much as granulated. It's so finely divided that it dissolves instantly and really hits your taste buds hard. It will help you feel like you're using a lot of sugar when you're not.

Oatmeal-Raisin Cookies

Ingredient	Amount to Make 16–24 Cookies
Breadspread	½ cup
Fructose	⅓ cup
Molasses	1 teaspoon
Vanilla	½ teaspoon
Egg substitute	⅔ cup (1 1/3 ounces)
Hodgson Mill whole wheat buttermilk pancake mix	½ cup
Cinnamon	¼ teaspoon
Old-fashioned or quick-cooking rolled oats	1 cup
Raisins	⅔ cup

Preheat oven to 350°. With a rubber spatula, mix breadspread and sugar. Add molasses, egg substitute, and vanilla and mix together. Mix all the dry ingredients in another small bowl, then add them to the mixture of wet ingredients. Mix till consistency is even. Spread in rounded tablespoonfuls on a cookie sheet sprayed with cooking spray or rubbed with a teaspoon of canola oil. Bake until the edges start to brown slightly. With a spatula, remove the cookies from the cookie sheet while they are hot. As soon as they are lukewarm, put them in an airtight container and seal it so they don't dry out.

1930's Carrot Cake

Balanced nutrition wasn't invented recently. This old recipe is updated only by substituting fructose for sugar. If you want it the truly authentic old-fashioned way, use a full cup of sugar instead.

Ingredient	Amount
Granulated fructose	½ cup
Raisins	1 cup
Grated carrots	1 ½ cups
Clove, ground	1 teaspoon
Water	1 ⅓ cup
Oil	2 tablespoons
Cinnamon	1 teaspoon
Nutmeg	1 teaspoon

Preheat oven to 350°. Boil all ingredients in a saucepan very slowly for 5 minutes. Cool to room temperature. Then add:

Walnuts	1 cup (optional)
Salt	pinch
Flour	2 cups
Baking soda	2 teaspoons

Mix till flour is just mixed in. Spread into a 9-inch pan and bake for 45 minutes, or spread into a 9-inch loaf pan and bake 1 ¼ hours.

Icing this cake is not necessary because it is so sweet and fruity. If your yen for cake includes icing, try this low-fat "buttercream" icing.

Buttercream Icing

Ingredient	Amount
Breadspread	1 tablespoon
Vanilla	½ teaspoon
Nonfat milk	½–1 teaspoon
Powdered sugar	½ cup

Mix the ingredients together in a small bowl with a fork. Add the smaller amount of milk until you see how thick or runny the icing is. For a firm cake or sweet rolls, the lesser amount is best, because it dries faster. For a soft cake (like carrot cake), the greater amount (or even more) is best, because the icing can be drizzled over the surface without tearing it. Makes enough to lightly ice a half-dozen sweet rolls or a small (8-inch by 8-inch) cake.

Slightly Exotic Apple Crisp

Skip the coriander and peanut butter (see below) for plain, down-home taste.

Filling Ingredient	Amount
Tart cooking apples	8 medium or 5–6 large
Granulated fructose	⅜ cup
or sugar or brown sugar	¾ cup
Ground cinnamon	1 teaspoon
Ground coriander	½ teaspoon
Ground nutmeg	½ teaspoon
Lemon juice	1 teaspoon or more to taste

Core apples; peel if desired. Slice apples in food processor. Pour into a 2-quart microwavable casserole. Add sugar and spices. Sprinkle with lemon. Stir with a big spoon.

Topping Ingredient	Amount
Rolled oats	¾ cup
Granulated fructose	⅜ cup
Ground cinnamon	1 teaspoon
Ground allspice	½ teaspoon
Peanut butter	1 tablespoon
Breadspread	2 tablespoons
Molasses	½ tablespoon

Stir ingredients together with a fork. When in sticky clumps, fork it over the filling. Bake in a 350° oven for 45 to 60 minutes, until apples are soft to an inserted fork (or microwave on High for 15 minutes). If 'waving and you want browning, broil for 3 to 5 minutes, watching for browning after the first 2 minutes—don't let it burn! Let cool at least 30 minutes. The slight tartness of vanilla frozen yogurt complements this dessert well.

Cheery All-Purpose Pie Crust

Ingredient	Amount
Multi-Grain Cheerios	½ cup of crumbs
Bread flour	1 cup
NuSalt or salt	½ teaspoon
Low-fat margarine or breadspread	4–5 ounces (see Chapter 14)

Crush Cheerios with a rolling pin between sheets of waxed paper, or use a blender. Mix all ingredients with a fork in a large bowl. Add margarine or breadspread until the mixture holds together when rolled between sheets of waxed paper. Roll the dough until it is about 12 inches in diameter. Press the rolled dough into a 9- or 10-inch pie pan. Dress up the edges by pressing crumb remnants onto the sides of the pan with dry hands. Bake at 350° for about 15 minutes, till crunchy.

Dutch Apple Pie

Make the all-purpose crust. Fill with the apple filling, add the topping, and bake as described for Apple Crisp.

Sweet Potato Pie

Filling Ingredient	Amount
Mashed cooked sweet potato or yam	1 ½ cups
Firmly packed brown sugar	½ cup
Optional: Molasses	½ teaspoon
and granulated fructose	¼ cup

Ground spices:

Pumpkin pie spice	½ tablespoon
or cinnamon	1 teaspoon
Allspice	½ teaspoon
Mace	¼ teaspoon
Optional: Finely chopped fresh ginger root	½ teaspoon

Salt or NuSalt	¾ teaspoon
Egg substitute	½ cup (equivalent to 2 eggs)
Nonfat evaporated milk	1 can (14½ ounces)
Margarine or breadspread	2 tablespoons

Mix all ingredients. Pour into a pie pan lined with pastry rolled ⅛-inch thick. (If using all-purpose pie crust, do not prebake it; just spray it with buttery-flavor cooking spray for 3 to 5 seconds before pouring on the filling). Bake in preheated oven at 425° for 10 minutes. Reduce heat to 350° and bake for 25 minutes or longer, until set. Cool before serving.

ℱRUIT COBBLERS

You can make cobblers two ways: with the biscuity dough on the top or on the bottom. Drop the filling on top and it's unmistakably a cobbler. Spread the crust on the bottom with a spatula, put the filling on top, and it bakes up to look a lot like a pie. Remember that, if the dough goes on top, it gets less of the juice in it. Either way, cobblers help you avoid the fat of a conventional pie crust and make a dessert that's more satisfying than pie. Use an 9- or 10-inch pie plate or an 8- or 9-inch casserole. The higher the sides, the less spilling into your oven.

Apple Cobbler Filling

Wash 7 large apples; cut off most of the skin and all the bruises. Thinly slice off all the goodie part of the apple, leaving the stems and core, into a big bowl holding a pint of water with 2 to 3 tablespoons of apple cider vinegar added. (The vinegar keeps the apples from turning brown.) After slicing in every apple, stir the bowl so all the apples are covered with vinegary water. Drain the sliced apples. Put them in the range-safe pie pan or casserole. Using your finger, mix 1 tablespoon of cornstarch and 1 teaspoon of cinnamon with 1 tablespoon of water till well dispersed. Add to ⅔ cup of apple cider. Stir. Pour over the sliced apples. Bring to a boil on the range and reduce to a simmer until apples are fork-soft (about 10 minutes); or bake at High in the microwave for 13 minutes.

Cherry Cobbler Filling

Drain one 15-ounce can of plain cherries for pie filling, reserving the juice. Put the cherries in a 2-quart saucepan. In a shallow, rounded cup, use your finger to mix 1 tablespoon of cornstarch and ½ teaspoon of cinnamon with 1 tablespoon of water till well dispersed. Add the suspension and ¼ cup of granulated fructose to the cherry juice. Stir. Pour over the cherries. Over medium heat, bring the mixture to a boil with constant stirring. Remove from heat as soon as the juice thickens; this should be within half a minute before or after it boils. If you like more tartness, add 1 tablespoon of dried or 2 tablespoon of fresh cranberries before heating the mixture to a boil.

Peach Cobbler Filling

Choose 6 to 9 peaches, depending on size. Peel, remove all bruises, and slice the peaches into a light plastic bowl to a total of a full pound. Toss the pits. Put the peaches in a 2-quart saucepan. Put 1 tablespoon of cornstarch and ½ teaspoon of cinnamon in a shallow, rounded cup. Using your finger, mix with 1 tablespoon of water till well dispersed. Add the suspension and ¼ cup of granulated fructose to ⅔ cup of peach beverage (After the Fall Georgia Peach or Knudsen's Peach Nectar). Stir. Pour over the peaches. Over medium heat, bring the mixture to a boil with constant stirring. Remove from heat as soon as the juice thickens; this should be within half a minute before or after it boils.

Cobbler Dough

Ingredient	Amount
Self-rising flour	⅔ cup
Brown sugar	¼ cup
Breadspread	2 tablespoons
Nonfat milk	¼–⅜ cup

Start with the minimum amount of milk. Mix with a fork for a few strokes, up to 25, just until the big lumps are gone. If the dough is not soft enough to drop in spoonfuls easily, add the rest of the milk and mix briefly. For a biscuity cobbler, drop the dough onto the precooked fruit filling. For a pie-like dessert, spread the dough into a pie plate with a rubber spatula, then put the precooked fruit filling on top. Bake at 350° for 25 to 30 minutes or until edges are golden brown.

Cobbler Toppings

Conventional cobblers are plain on top, with their biscuits showing, but no one can stop you from adding a topping if you want to. Here are a few suggestions:

Pecans. Mix about 2 tablespoons of crushed pecans with 1 tablespoon of granulated fructose or brown sugar and 1/2 teaspoon of cinnamon, apple pie spice, or pumpkin pie spice. Sprinkle over cobbler with a spoon before baking.

Oaty Crunch

Ingredient	Amount
Rolled oats (regular or 1-minute)	¼ cup
Granulated fructose or brown sugar	¼ cup
Breadspread	2 tablespoons
Flour	1 tablespoon

You can substitute granola (without fruit) for the oats. Mix all ingredients with a fork in a small bowl. Fork the mix over the cobbler before baking.

Fruity or Other Extra-Flavorful Yogurt

Commercial fruit yogurts are panned nutritionally, even though yogurt itself is wonderful for you. Why the criticism? Because a cup of commercial fruit yogurt has only about 90 calories worth of yogurt, but 22 to over 60 calories worth of butterfat, and about 160 calories (40 grams) of sugar. Sure, it tastes sweet enough. But do you need all that sugar? Do you want it? Instead, try the following mix, using Dannon or another good brand of yogurt—one that is thick instead of runny and has no gelatin in it. If your plain yogurt has liquid on top (whey), pour it off before you use it.

Ingredient	Amount
Plain nonfat yogurt	4–6 ounces
Polaner or other all-fruit spread	1 tablespoon
Honey	1 overflowing teaspoon
Vanilla	1 teaspoon

Mix ingredients. Rechill for an hour if you want it even thicker. Sprinkle with ½ teaspoon of granulated fructose and a pinch of cinnamon, allspice, or apple pie spice, if desired. Peach or apricot goes well with a teaspoon of crushed walnuts.

Don't want fruit? Make the recipe without the fruit spread, or substitute ½ teaspoon of freeze-dried coffee, heated and stirred with 1 teaspoon of granulated fructose and 1 tablespoon of water. Add your favorite addition for coffee, too—a sprinkling of cinnamon, perhaps.

Frozen Yogurt

Ice cream-makers are fine for making homemade frozen yogurt. What it lacks in the smoothness of commercial frozen yogurt, it makes up in fresher taste.

MAKING

The recipes for fruity or other extra-flavorful yogurt are a good starting point. Make a volume half of that recommended for your ice cream maker. Then, so it's not amazingly sour, add the same volume of 1 percent milk. (Skim milk tends to make a disagreeably thin, icy frozen dessert). Also, you are likely to find that the sweet taste of sugar or honey tends to get lost when it is frozen. So add more honey or sugar than is already in the mixture of yogurt and milk, up to ½ to ⅔ the amount of sugar recommended in the recipe book that comes with your ice cream maker, or the same volume of honey. Then process the mix as per your ice cream maker's directions.

SERVING

Serve immediately for that soft-serve freshness. If you prefer hard frozen desserts, put the frozen yogurt in your freezer for at least 2 hours before serving. If the frozen yogurt isn't sweet enough, add a sweetened topping or put unfrozen (sweeter) fruit on top. Didn't you want a sundae, anyway?

If you want to make small servings, pour the soft frozen yogurt into ice cube trays and add popsicle sticks before it freezes hard. To serve, flip the tray over, run it under a *little* warm water, and ease the yogurtsicle out by the stick handle.

For fanciness or to return yogurt-sicles to frozen storage: Dredge in a mixture of 5 parts fructose to 1 part ground cinnamon. Bag the 'sicles you won't eat immediately, and return them to the freezer. Coated yogurt-sicles won't stick together.

Fruit Salad

Fruit salad needs a proper mixture of sweet and sour, firm pieces and crunchy bits, and lots of different shapes and colors for variety and interest. Add a bit of juice to help keep it moist. Use whatever fruit is your favorite, but avoid citrus to help your stomach. Preservatives make commercial fruit salad taste terrible. Use up the salad while it's fresh.

Sweet: grapes, ripe banana slices, Delicious apple chunks, peach bits, slices of ripe or canned pear, raisins, pineapple bits, honeydew melon balls, cantaloupe bits, or watermelon balls. Tangerine or mandarin orange have so much sweetness and so little acid that they may not hurt your stomach; try a small amount to test.

Tart: tart cherries, unripe banana slices, unripe pears, Granny Smith or other tart apple slices, fresh strawberries, blueberries, raspberries, or star fruit slices. All these sour fruits should have too little acid to hurt you. When in doubt, eat only small amounts.

Crunchy or chewy: dried fruit pieces—cherries, cranberries, apricots, etc.—or fresh coconut or nutmeats. Use fresh coconut meat. Cut it in small bits; it's chock-full of saturated fat. Nutmeats are high in fat also, but have little or no saturated fat; use them sparingly.

Exotic: Mango slices (strong taste; use sparingly), papaya.

Part 4

MORE ON MEDICINE

Chapter 23

WHAT THE DOCTOR CAN DO FOR YOU

$\mathcal{I}$f you're under the age of 45 and you have chronic, mild symptoms of intestinal or stomach distress, most gastroenterologists will begin by recommending nonmedical changes. Topping the list are diet, exercise, and avoidance of smoking and alcohol.

Some symptom patterns point to a need for doctoring. One is belly pain that goes away after eating. This usually signals peptic ulcer disease.

Dyspepsia during anti-inflammatory drug use (see sidebar) means serious stomach problems. This happens frequently, so you'll need a doctor to sort out the possibilities. Also, *alarm symptoms* such as weight loss, trouble swallowing, or anemia need special care. And anyone over the age of 45 who has new dyspepsia should have a doctor's workup.

The reason to go to a doctor for such symptoms is not just that they don't improve without doctoring; sometimes they do spontaneously disappear. The real reason to see a doctor is that these illnesses frequently lead to bleeding, perforation, or even cancer. If that's what's happening, you want to catch the problem as early as possible. Stomach and esophageal cancers are among those with the worst survival rates, because they are usually discovered too late.

If you have any of the symptoms that are known as "alarm signals," your doctor can run the necessary tests and provide the medications or treatments that you need. Ultimately, of course, it would be ideal to achieve healing without medications or surgery. That's not always possible. But your doctor can probably suggest ways that good medicine can be combined with lifestyle changes to produce the best possible results.

ARE YOU HAVING "ALARM SYMPTOMS?"

In Japan, stomach cancer occurs more frequently than in the U.S. population. To help people identify warning symptoms, Japanese gastroenterologists have identified a list of "alarm symptoms." While these symptoms don't mean that you have stomach cancer, they indicate that you should definitely see a doctor—preferably a gastroenterologist—for a thorough examination, particularly if you have weight loss, anemia, or jaundice.

SYMPTOM OR SIGN	SEE A PHYSICIAN IF
Appetite loss or weight loss	You lose 7 pounds or more without trying, or if you don't eat unless urged by others.
Anemia	You're weak and pale and don't know why.
Difficulty swallowing	Swallowed food hurts or "hangs up" in the chest.
Jaundice	Eyes or skin turn yellow.
History of ulcer or cancer; strong family history of cancer	You develop dyspepsia ("stomach ache") or other new symptoms of intestinal distress.
Current use of NSAID* drugs	Dyspepsia occurs.
GI bleeding	You vomit "coffee grounds" or blood, or you have black or red stools in your bowel movements.
Worsening of pain induced by eating high-fat foods or drinking alcohol	The pain lasts for an hour on 2 days in a row or on more than 1 day per week.

*Non-steroid anti-inflammatory drugs: ibuprofen, aspirin, etc.

Don't assume that a worse or more frequent kind of discomfort is from the same old mild ailment you have always had. Some ulcers are malignant rather than benign. So are some swallowing difficulties. And many a belly pain originates in an organ other than the stomach. If you don't get expert diagnosis, changing your diet and hoping for a safe outcome may hurt you rather than help you.

SYMPTOM OR SIGN	SEE A PHYSICIAN IF
Localized pain with pressure	Your belly is tender to the touch.
Failure of several treatments	Self-treatment with lifestyle changes, antacids, or acid blockers for two weeks has failed.

People's weight may fluctuate. Women, in particular, may lose more than 7 pounds in a month. But if you lose that much, you should have some clear and obvious explanation (such as that you've been on a strict diet). Otherwise, see your doctor.

Anemia means low concentrations of red blood cells in the blood. It can come from vitamin deficiencies, but the usual and worrisome cause is from significant, chronic blood loss. You need to see your doctor if you have anemia, because that blood loss could be occurring in the gastrointestinal tract.

Jaundice is yellowing of the skin that comes from disease of the liver. This is related to your gastrointestinal system because a special group of veins, called the hepatic portal system, collects whatever passes out of the lining of the entire upper-GI tract and conducts it to the liver. The hepatic portal system also channels to the liver whatever cells break loose from the esophagus, stomach, and small intestine, and the sieve-like liver entraps them. So the liver is the first organ likely to be invaded by a cancer that originates in other organs in the gastrointestinal system.

You may need much more than a dietary change—you might need surgery or prescription medication. There has been a revolution in medical care of serious stomach ailments, so avail yourself of the opportunity to benefit from the treatments that are now available.

In this chapter, I offer some guidelines and tips for working with your doctor to get the maximum benefit from the holistic healing approaches and the diet and lifestyle changes that I have already described in this book. Here's what you'll find in this part:

➦ What to do before you see a gastroenterologist

➦ What to expect during an examination

➦ What the doctor is looking for

In Chapter 24, we'll discuss:

➦ Possible medications and treatments

➦ Possible side effects from various medications, and what to do about them

Let's begin with your visit to the doctor.

$\mathcal{W}$HAT TO DO BEFORE YOU SEE A GASTROENTEROLOGIST

Most doctors recommend that you keep a diary to help with the diagnosis. For two weeks to a month, write down what symptoms you get, when they hit, how long they last, and what relieves them or makes them worse. Make a note of any medications you're taking—including over-the-counter medicines like aspirin or antihistamines—and also the food and beverages in your daily diet.

At the end of each day, track your symptoms: what you felt, when, for how long, and how intense the symptoms were. The doctor will best understand three intensity terms: Use "mild" if the symptom annoys but does not get in your way enough to slow you down or require immediate treatment. Use "moderate" if the symptom does slow you down or partially prevents you from engaging in any activities or requires immediate treatment, say with antacid tablets. (Did it nag and distract you from work?) Use "severe" if it prevents activities. (Did it make you go rest?).

Also write down in the diary how you treated the symptoms. How many Rolaids® or swallows of Mylanta® did you take, at what time? Did you bend over and hold your stomach awhile? Bounce up and down and make yourself belch? Drink some milk or other cold fluid, just to ease pain? Did it help or make the symptoms disappear entirely? How long did that take?

Write down what you took in before the trouble began. Don't write an essay on every food and beverage you take every day; just write down what you ate or drank within a couple of hours before any trouble began. Or, if you ate nothing, write down for how many hours you were fasting. Don't forget to write down all the beverages in this critical time period.

While we're on the subject of "things you took in," include any stresses in the same period. Angry words from the spouse? New demands from the boss? Noticed that you were running late? A problem with one of the children? No distractions, so you started worrying about a problem? Any other straw that broke the camel's back—anything, big or not, that "made" you upset?

We're not *blaming* here. The idea is neither to pin a problem on somebody else nor to make you feel guilty or ridiculous about your own reactions. The object is simply to understand what leads to your distress.

It's important to quantify stress. So estimate, each day, how much time you spent being upset or worrying, or doing something excessive—anything nonproductive—to ward off or undo distress. Include rituals such as cleaning, straightening, and rechecking. Include TV-watching if it's done to avoid distress. Apply the intensity labels here too: Was your reaction mild, moderate, or severe?

$\mathcal{W}$HAT TO EXPECT DURING AN EXAMINATION

When you tell a doctor about stomach symptoms, the doctor will begin right away to decide what you *don't* have and try to figure out what you *do* have. In the process of doing this (called a differential diagnosis), the doctor will begin checking off a variety of possibilities. Do you have heartburn? Ulcer? Gastritis? Do your symptoms suggest esophageal reflux?

These are just a few of the possibilities, ranging in seriousness from minor to severe. First, the doctor has to find out what the main symptom is. Is it pain? If so, when during the day does the pain occur? How is that pain related to food?

Is the main problem a symptom like weight loss or anemia (the lack of energy that results from having a low count of red blood cells)? Do you have trouble swallowing? Is the pain worse after you've been eating? Does your stomach feel tender? Do you have blood in your stool?

If the gastroenterologist decides to give you an internal examination, the doctor may want to "scope" you. This means passing a flexible endoscope into your stomach to look directly at what's going on and make the diagnosis.

The endoscopy procedure is actually called esophagogastroduodenoscopy, or EGD. During the procedure, the doctor looks at the lining of the esophagus, stomach, and duodenum (the first short bend of the small intestine past the stomach).

This technology required the invention of fiber optics in the 1950s. The endoscope is a long, flexible tube about as big around as a finger. It has three tiny appliances at the end that goes toward the stomach: a pincer to take biopsy samples, a flashlight, and an objective lens. The operator's end has controls for the pincer and light plus a receptacle for interchangeable optics—an eyepiece to look through, connection to a TV monitor, and a Polaroid or 35 mm camera body. In between is a cable of fiber optics.

It's not hard to take being endoscoped because of the preparation the doctor gives. A strong but short-acting sedative is given, usually as a shot, plus a spray that numbs the throat. The sedative leaves the patient just conscious enough to sit and cooperate. Also, the procedure is mercifully short, taking only a few minutes.

$\mathcal{W}$HAT THE DOCTOR IS LOOKING FOR

If pain is the predominant complaint, and you notice that the pain disappears whenever you're eating, this usually means peptic ulcer. There are many successful ways to treat peptic ulcer, and it should be treated as soon as possible. An ulcer is like a raw, open wound in the stomach. If left untreated, the wound can go all the way through the stomach wall, causing severe inflammation, or through blood vessels, causing bleeding.

Peptic ulcer in the stomach itself may not produce typical ulcer symptoms. In fact, it's sometimes caused by nothing more than pain-relief medications.

A peptic ulcer can also occur in the *duodenum*, the uppermost part of the small intestine, which directly receives the outflow of acidic contents from the stomach. If that's where it is, the pain is sharp and noticeable. In other words, you really *feel* the ulcer in the duodenum, whereas if you have one in the stomach, the pain is less detectable.

"Scoping" may show no ulcer as a cause of long-term stomach pain, but instead a pattern of superficial erosions. This is *chronic active gastritis*, and it needs treatment too.

If the pain occurs at any time of day, but especially after eating, that's *non-ulcer dyspepsia*, which means you'll have heartburn symptoms. What causes it? Nothing but backwash of acid from the stomach up into the esophagus. This can burn the lower esophagus, cause trouble swallowing, and even lead to cancer. So even though heartburn is very common, these symptoms are not to be ignored.

Heartburn occurs when the *lower esophageal sphincter* (the LES) fails. This is a ring of muscles that is supposed to keep the acid down in the stomach. Smoking, stress, strains such as bending over, and certain drugs and foods weaken the ring.

Heartburn, as far too many of us know, is the nagging central chest pain that occurs after eating, especially after bending over or straining or belching. It may be accompanied by a sour taste in the back of the mouth. The sour taste (sometimes just a food taste or a watery sensation) may occur after eating even if you don't feel the pain of heartburn. Regurgitation produces all of this, just as when a baby spits up when burped.

Fifteen million Americans get heartburn daily. The good news is that a quarter of those with symptoms severe enough to indicate reflux esophagitis—inflammation—have normal esophageal biopsies, and fewer than 20 percent have acute inflammatory changes. To translate that, it means that heartburn may cause no further problem at all. But sometimes it *does*, and that's why your doctor will want you to keep track of it.

Heartburn comes from backwash of stomach contents into the esophagus. This is basting the strongest acid in the body onto an organ that is not designed to withstand it. It hurts, of course; your lower esophagus is receiving a mild chemical burn. That irritation of the esophageal lining, its mucosa, frequently can inflame it, causing a condition that doctors name *reflux esophagitis*.

When inflammation of the "skin" of the esophagus occurs chronically, it can kill the cells, the *mucosa*. An array of flattened, tile-like cells gets replaced by rod-like cells that are packed together upright. (In medical language, squamous epithelium, comprised of flattened cells, is replaced by columnar epithelium, the rod-like cells.)

Doctors take notice, because this condition, called Barrett's esophagus, is a risk factor for developing esophageal cancer. Barrett's occurs in 10 to 15 percent of those with chronic heartburn. Those who have this precancerous change have a risk of cancer over 40 times higher than that of the general population.

The burning can reach deeper, too, causing inflammation of the deeper layers of the esophagus. This or the scarring that follows from it can be severe enough to cause *stricture*. Stricture means tightening of the tissue, and when that occurs, you'll have trouble swallowing (dysphagia). Other signs that heartburn is worsening are pain on swallowing hot and cold foods, or pain on swallowing slightly acid foods.

There is no medical dividing line between recurrent or chronic heartburn and what's called *gastroesophageal reflux disease* (GERD). Scoping and, especially, a brief test period of treatment tell the doctor how aggressively to proceed in further treatment of the problem.

Often GERD is caused by a hiatus hernia. This is an upward bulge of the stomach that protrudes up through the normal hole (hiatus) in the diaphragm. Rarely, surgery may be necessary for the hiatus, but the usual treatment for GERD with a hiatus hernia is the same as if there were no hiatus hernia—that is, lifestyle management and medications. The combination should be tried for up to two weeks.

OTHER SIGNS OF MEDICAL PROBLEMS

Abdominal pain with pressure is usually something a doctor finds during a physical exam; it's pain on pressing fingers into the abdomen. If the pain during palpation, called tenderness, is limited to one small area of the belly (point tenderness), that's a sign of a diseased organ.

If the tenderness is not localized, or if there is generalized abdominal pain without tenderness, the doctor may suspect irritable bowel syndrome (IBS) or low-grade food allergies. Neither are the subject of this book, but they are frequent and chronic. They are also highly treatable, though treatment may require a clinical ecologist M.D., a naturopath, or some other holistic practitioner.

The doctor is sure to ask you about other symptoms as well. Do you ever vomit blood? Have you detected any blood in your stool when you have bowel movements?

GI bleeding can be grossly visible as bloody vomitus (hematemesis) or stools (hematochezia). More often, vomiting associated with a bleeding stomach looks like coffee grounds, because of the effects of stomach acid on the blood.

Stool, too, more often looks black than red from upper-GI tract bleeding, for the same reason. These black stools are called melena.

Still more often, there is no trace of black, and blood is found only when the stool is sent to the lab for what's called a "chemical stool blood test." The generic version is called a stool guaiac test; the usual brand-name test is the Hematest. None of these tests is proof positive; no chemical test is that good. They all miss a goodly fraction of GI bleeding, and so they must be repeated several times.

Worsening of pain after eating high-fat foods or drinking alcohol, especially in large quantities, alerts the clinician to problems in other organs—the gallbladder and pancreas, respectively.

Chapter 24

$\mathcal{M}$EDICATIONS AND TREATMENTS THAT CAN HELP YOUR STOMACH

$\mathcal{G}$astroenterologists have a wide range of prescription medications that can help you, and that's another good reason for seeing the doctor for any serious or alarming stomach symptoms.

Specific prescription medications have a high rate of "cure" for peptic ulcer and for controlling GERD and chronic active gastritis, especially the medications that have been developed since the 1970s. Many of these medications slow down the flow of stomach acid rather than attacking the root cause of the ulcer. Even so, they can be effective.

Nowadays, the top choice among these is the group called proton pump inhibitors. Prilosec®, the first of them, is the biggest-selling prescription drug in the world, and for good reason! It can heal almost any ulcer. It shuts down the secretion of acid by the stomach.

Since Prilosec®, other effective medications have also been® introduced. Prevacid® (lasoprazole, TAP), Aciphex® (rabeprazole), Protonix® (pantoprazole), and Nexium® (esomeprazole) are equally effective competitors.

Histamine-type 2 receptor antagonists (H_2 blockers) such as Tagamet® and Zantac® led the way before Prilosec®. They're still good at healing ulcers and treating heartburn, especially at night. They are not as powerful by day, though, and can produce side effects. Other H_2 blockers include Merck's Pepcid® and Lilly's Axid®. The FDA found all four of these drugs so safe as to allow sale of them over-the-counter, although at half the prescription dosage per pill. This amount should not be enough to treat a full-fledged ulcer without taking quite a few doses a day. However, the concentrations sold in over-the-counter formulas are enough to treat simple heartburn or an upset stomach about two-thirds of the time.

The real cause of peptic ulcer seems to be a microbe. Eradicating it with antibiotics cures the ulcer, and for a longer time than acid blockers do. But many people carry the "bug," *Helicobacter pylori*, in their stomachs without getting ulcers. With the proper combination of antibiotics, the recurrence of peptic ulcer (in a 38-week period) was reduced from 95 percent to 12 percent!

The ulcer microbe is so hardy that it may take a triple-threat offense using antibiotics to kill it and cure the ulcer. But as the tests show, results are impressive. There's a problem with antibiotics, however. If you take them for an extended time, even under a doctor's close supervision, antibiotics can cause major side effects. And treatment with antibiotics is only the short-term story. Over 15 years of follow-up, it has been found that the incidence of peptic ulcer is twice as great in people who face serious life stresses. So total reliance on a doctor's medication, instead of exercising some self-reliance on reducing stress, is not the whole answer.

Additional drugs recommended for treating other upper GI problems, such as GERD, are usually a prokinetic agent, an H_2 blocker, or an antacid.

Prokinetic drugs make the contractions of the esophageal sphincter, the stomach, and the intestine work better. The only one now available in the United States is Reglan®, which can cause major side effects but is also dramatically effective in healing the esophagus.

The second medical treatment option is H_2 blockers or antacids. Backwash without acid is benign to the esophagus, so acid blockers and antacids—over-the-counter agents—can relieve the problem too.

ᴡHAT ABOUT ANTACIDS?

Antacids are a few of the last surviving drugs that do not work on any receptor in the body. This means they have little reserve power. They mainly neutralize the acid that is present when they are taken. That's the real meaning behind "How do you spell relief?" They can help for a short time only, providing relief rather than continuing benefit.

What happens next is a new ballgame, almost totally dependent on the stomach. A high dose (e.g., a full ounce of a liquid antacid such as Mylanta® or six of the chewable tablets) can give protection against later acid outflow for up to two hours. The usual dose of 1 or 2 tablets gives an hour of protection or less. All are fairly promptly evacuated to the small intestine, where they have no efficacy.

Antacids are carbonates, so they absorb stomach acid (protons, really hydrogen ions) and, in doing so, form carbonic acid. Carbonic acid is unstable in water and partially releases water and carbon dioxide. Thus, the natural outcome of taking carbonate antacids to relieve hyperacidity is bloating and belching. This is not the best result, because the (partially) neutralized stomach contents can then splash up into the esophagus.

Some antacids are aluminum or calcium carbonates, which can cause constipation. Others are magnesium carbonates, which can cause diarrhea. Some antacids are a mix of both a binding and a loosening carbonate to minimize bowel side effects.

Aluminum is slightly absorbable, and it can interfere with bone metabolism and possibly affect other organs. So taking aluminum carbonates chronically is not necessarily benign. Antacids may also interact with some drugs, binding them from being absorbed.

Tums® touts its calcium content because of recent findings that 1000 or even 1500 mg of elemental calcium a day can help prevent bone deterioration and fractures. Calcium is not well absorbed from a salt as simple as calcium carbonate. (See Chapter 10, Minerals by the Gram.)

One antacid is different, Gaviscon®. It floats on the surface of the stomach contents, neutralizing the part that could otherwise damage the esophagus on regurgitation. Clinical research with careful measurement of acidity has shown that Gaviscon® keeps the pH (acidity) much more nearly neutral up at the gastroesophageal junction for two hours after a dose.

A number of antacids contain simethicone, an "anti-gas" agent. Simethicone does not prevent formation of gas or neutralize it in any way, but it does break up bubbles of gas. Whether this helps to expel it from the body is unclear.

Whatever antacid one takes, the dose for relief of GERD (if it has been prescribed by a physician) is an ounce of the regular-strength liquid or 4 to 6 tablets of the regular-strength tablets; or a tablespoon of double-strength liquid or up to 4 tablets of double-strength tablets. The regimen required is a dose two hours after every meal and every two hours until the next meal.

Chapter 25

ᗩRE MEDICINES OR SUPPLEMENTS *HURTING* YOUR STOMACH?

𝒟rugs that are most used as pain relievers, called NSAID for Non-Steroidal Anti-Inflammatory Drugs (see sidebar), are the biggest cause of stomach erosions and ulcers. These medicines include aspirin, ibuprofen (Advil®, Nuprin®, Motrin®, and other brands), naproxen (Anaprox®, Naprosyn®, Releve®), ketoprofen (Orudis®, Orudis KT®) and many brands available only on prescription, such as Indocin®, Lodine®, Relafen®, and Voltaren®.

Many combinations of aspirin or ibuprofen with other drugs are also marketed over the counter, so read labels if you are still in doubt about whether any medicine you take contains an NSAID.

Not all NSAIDs are created equal. The most common one, ibuprofen, is the safest one for the stomach, at least at low doses. Those with highest risk, Toradol® (ketorolac) and Ponstel® (mefamanic acid), are not for chronic use. Aspirin is so ulcerogenic that taking only 3 tablets a day (1 gram) increases the risk of hospitalization for ulcer tenfold. In chronic use, the relative risk of an ulcer complication, compared to ibuprofen, is highest with an NSAID called azapropazone (Rheumox® or Tolyprin®, not available in the U.S.), more than ten times the risk of ibuprofen. The risk is three- to fivefold with ketoprofen (Orudis®), piroxicam (Feldene®), and tolmetin (Tolectin®); two- to threefold with indomethacin (Indocin®), naproxen (Naprosyn®, Anaprox®, Aleve®), diflunisal (Dolobid®),sulindac (Clinoril®), and diclofenac (Voltaren®, Cataflam®); and about twofold with aspirin and fenoprofen (Nalfon®).

PAIN RELIEF . . . AT A COST

Here are the NSAIDs (non-steroidal anti-inflammatory drugs) that can contribute to stomach or intestinal problems. If you are taking any of these, be sure to let your doctor know. There may be a substitute that will work just as well (or better!) without causing the side effects that hurt your stomach.

GENERIC NAME	BRAND NAMES	
	PRESCRIPTION	OVER-THE-COUNTER
Ibuprofen	Motrin®, IBU®, others and in combinations	Advil®, Motrin IB®, Nuprine®, etc. and in combinations
Indomethacin	Indocin®	
Naproxen	Naprosyn®, Anaprox®	Releve®
Oxaprozin	Daypro®	
Ketoprofen	Orudis®	Orudis KT®
Sulindac	Clinoril®	
Diflunisal	Dolobid®	
Piroxicam	Feldene®	
Flurbiprofen	Ansaid®	
Diclofenac	Cataflam®, Voltaren®	
Flurbiprofen	Ansaid®	
Fenoprofen	Nalfon®	
Mefanamic acid	Ponstel®	
Nabumetone	Relafen®	
Ketorolac	Toradol®	
Tolmetin	Tolectin®	
Etodolac	Lodine®	

NSAIDs bother some of us more than others, depending (among other things) on your age, your sex, and the dose you take. If you're over 60, you have a higher risk of having an adverse reaction to NSAIDs. Women are at greater risk than men. And for all groups, the risk of side effects is worse if you take higher doses. The British found ibuprofen extremely benign when it was first marketed in the 1970s, but they restricted dosage to 200 milligrams at a time, with 800 milligrams as a maximum daily total. Now, some doctors prescribe ibuprofen tablets that are two, three, or even four times as potent. As a result, ibuprofen is recognized as sometimes ulcerogenic—that is, it can cause ulcers.

Do not take these precautions lightly. The NSAIDs cause at least 60 percent of complicated ulcers (those with hemorrhage or perforation).

The newest NSAIDs—Daypro® (oxaprozen), Relafen® (nabumetone), and Lodine® (etodolac)—were produced specifically to lower this risk, and with partial success. Yet good old ibuprofen remains the lowest-risk NSAID in some large population studies.

The new COX-2 inhibitors promise to reduce the risk further. Yet, reports of ulcers and bleeding have jumped alarmingly with some of these drugs since their marketing in Europe. Merck's COX-2 inhibitor is Vioxx® (rofecoxib) and Searle's is Celebrex® (celecoxib). A third one, Boehringer Ingelheim's Mobic® (meloxicam), has just been approved. Call it a COX-and-a-half; its risk may be intermediate between the older drugs and the COX-2 agents.

Why not avoid all of the stomach risk and substitute Tylenol® (acetaminophen)? Tylenol® simply does not cause ulcer or bleeding. But it is modestly effective for pain and minimally anti-inflammatory, even at large doses. And there is a definite ceiling on the daily dosage that can be used, or else the risk of liver toxicity increases.

If you need an NSAID and you are at risk for developing ulcers, ask your doctor to work out a program to substitute some of it with acetaminophen—or all of it during easier periods. If 1000 milligrams at a time, three times a day or less, works for you, you can get all of the benefit with acetaminophen, with none of the risk to the liver.

Use of multiple anti-inflammatory drugs at the same time, particularly adding a corticosteroid such as prednisone to an NSAID, increases the risk of ulcer.

Finally, of course, having had an ulcer in the past renders one more likely to get a new one when taking an NSAID.

𝒯HE RISK OF MIXING DRUGS

There is a long list of other medicines that often cause dyspepsia. Everyone with dyspepsia should be alert to these drugs as potentially causing their problems. One warning before you find a culprit and say, "Aha! I'm getting rid of that @# today!" **Don't stop any prescription medicines just because you see them on this list!**

Your medicine was prescribed for an important reason, so don't just stop it on your own. Call your doctor, get an appointment, and ask for a substitute that's easier on the stomach. Tell—or remind—your doctor what your stomach symptoms are. And go to the appointment armed with a few days of diary entries showing whether the symptoms arise regularly after taking the medicine.

Poring over this list is not necessarily going to identify your problem. After heading a large pharmaceutical company's adverse reaction department for a few years, I had to conclude that any drug can cause any reaction, at least rarely. So the question for you is, regardless of this list or any other, does your particular biochemistry disagree with any medicine you take, even if that drug does not cause dyspepsia in most other people? If you are concerned about the relation between any medicine you take and stomach symptoms, tell your doctor and ask for a substitute.

꿏꒞ꓹꜟꜙ

PRESCRIPTION MEDICINES THAT OFTEN CAUSE DYSPEPSIA

This is a list of drugs that *frequently* causes dyspepsia symptoms. This list is from a recent edition of the *Physician's Desk Reference*, but it's not totally complete. Be sure to tell your doctor about *any* medications you're taking. There are some that only occasionally cause stomach pain, nausea, or gastritis—but you might be one of the people who are affected that way.

	NAMES	
DRUG CLASS	**GENERIC**	**BRAND**
Antibiotics in chronic use (e.g., for acne)	Erythromycin	A/T/S®, E.E.S.®, E-mycin®, Erytabs®, Erythrocin®
	Minocycline	Minocin®
	Doxycycline	Vibramycin®
Cancer Chemotherapy	Paclitaxel	Taxol®
	Methotrexate	
	Most others	
Corticosteroids	Betamethasone	Celestone®
	Cortisone	Cortone®
	Dexamethasone	Decadron®
	Hydrocortisone	Hydrocortone®
	Methylpredinosolone	Medrol®
	Prednisone	Deltasone®
	Prednisolone	Prelone®
	Triamcinolone	Aristocort®
Analgesics, opioid-type	Butorphanol	Stadol®
	Codeine	Empirin® with Codeine, No. 3 and No. 4, many others
	Fentanyl	Duragesic®
	Morphine	MS Contin®, MS IR®, Oramorph SR®, Roxanol®
	Oxycodone	OxyContin® Percocet®, Percogesic®, Percodan®, Tylox®

DRUG CLASS	NAME	
	GENERIC	BRAND
	Hydrocodone	Lortabs®, Lorcet®, Vicodin®
	Meperidine	Demerol®
	Pentazocine	Talacen®, Talwin Nx®
	Tramadol	Ultram®
Alzheimer's disease management drugs	Tacrine	Cognex®
	Donepezil	Aricept®
Anti-abusive drugs	Naltrexone	ReVia®
	Disulfiram	Antabuse® (alcohol, shave lotion or vinegars can cause reaction)
Antidepressants and mood stabilizers	Lithium	Eskalith®, Lithobid®
	Clomipramine	Anafranil®
	Nefazodone	Serzone®
	Fluoxetine	Prozac®
	Paroxetine	Paxil®
	Sertraline	Zoloft®
	Fluvoxamine	Luvox®
	Venlafaxine	Effexor®
Anti-anxiety drugs	Buspirone	BuSpar®
Anti-rheumatoid drugs	Hydroxychloroquin Plaquenil Methotrexate	
Calcemic agents	Fosamax! Etidronate	Didronel® (when taken at 10–20 mg/day, not 5 mg)

DRUG CLASS	NAME	
	GENERIC	**BRAND**
Cardiovascular	Digoxin	Lanoxin®
	Niacin	
	Quinidine	Quinidex®, Quinaglute®
	Procainamide	Pronestyl®, Procan SR®, Procanbid®
	Fluvastatin	Lescol®
	Lovastatin	Mevacor®
	Pravastatin	Pravachol®
	Simvastatin	Zocor®
Anti-Parkinsonism drugs	Bromocriptine	Parlodel®
	Carbidopa-levodopa	Sinemet®, Atamet®
	Levodopa	Larodopa®
	Pergolide	Permax®
	Pramipexole	Mirapex®
Anti-epileptic drugs	Carbamazepine	Atretol®, Tegretol®
	Felbamate	Felbatol®
Mineral supplements	Potassium	K-Dur®, K-Lor®, K-Lyte®, Slow-K®, K-Tab®, K-Phos®, Klor-Con®
Anti-asthmatic	Theophylline	Marax®, Quibron®, Mudrane®, Theolate®, Slo- bid®, Slo-Phyllin®, Aerolate®, Theo-24®, Theo-Dur®, Uni-Dur®, Uniphyl®, Theoclear®, Theolair®

SUPPLEMENTS THAT CAN SABOTAGE YOU

Some dietary supplements can also cause stomach distress. Just because someone at the health food store recommends a supplement doesn't mean that it's bound to be good for you in particular. We are each unique. So be sure to notice what happens after you take any of these supplements.

STIMULANTS	IRRITANTS	OTHERS
Oil in Large Quantity (>1 tbsp. at a time)	Saw Palmetto	Multivitamins
Fish Oil	Cayenne, Jalapeno, other peppers	Carnitine, other amino amino acids
Laxatives: Cascara, Gentian, Barberry	Mustard	Comfrey for long periods of time
Nuts	Hydrochloric acid	Enzymes (if stomach is already irritated)
Caffeine	Niacin!	Zinc
Spices	Vinegar	Dong Qai
	Ascorbic acid (>250 mg at a time)	

ꟿEDICINES THAT BOTHER THE LES

While we know that heartburn is caused by failure of the lower esophogeal sphincter or LES, we don't yet understand why that trap door between the stomach and the lower esophagus can so often fail. Certain foods can weaken the LES, and, as I've noted, you should try to stay away from chocolate, fat, peppermint, alcohol, and caffeine if you have heartburn. Stopping them can be of great help.

In addition, however, there are a dozen different common types of drugs that can weaken the LES (see sidebar). Most of these are prescription drugs that are important for treating other conditions. Be sure to talk to your doctor about possible alternatives.

DRUGS THAT WEAKEN THE LOWER ESOPHAGEAL SPHINCTER

CLASS OF DRUGS	EXAMPLES (TRADE NAMES)
Central analgesics (opioids)	Morphine®, (MS Contin®, Roxanol®), Oxycodone (OxyContin®, Tylox®), Meperidine (Demerol®) etc.*
Muscle relaxants	Diazepam (Valium®), Cyclobenzaprine (Flexeril®). Possibly methocarbamol Robaxin®), carisoprodol (Soma®), Metaxolon (Skelaxin®) and/or Chlorzoxazone (Parafon Forte®).
Barbiturate sedatives	Phenobarbital (Nembutal®), Secobarbital (Seconal®), Butalbital (Phrenillin®)
Anticholinergic drugs for colds, motion sickness, urinary incontinence, ulcer	Belladonna (atropine, scopolamine, Donnatal®, Transderm Scop®, Urised®), Dicyclomine (Bentyl®), Flavoxate (Urispas®), Hyoscyamine (Cystospaz®, Levbid®, Levsin®), Oxybutynin (Ditropan®)
Tricyclic antidepressants	Imipramine (Tofranil®), Amitriptyline (Elavil®), Desipramine (Norpramin®), Doxepin (Sinequan®, Adapin®) Clomipramine (Anafranil®), others
Phenothiazine antipsychotic drugs	Chlorpromazine (Thorazine®), Thioridazine (Mellaril®), Promethazine (Phenergan®), Prochlorperazine (Compazine®), Trifluoperazine (Stelazine®), others
Calcium channel blockers (for high blood pressure, cardiac pain, and some other cardiovascular indications)	Amlodipine (Norvasc®), Bepridil (Vascor®), Diltiazem (Cardizem®, Dilacor®), Felodipine (Plendil®), Nifedipine (Adalat®, Procardia®), Nimodepine (Nimotop®), Isradapine (Dynacirc®), Nicardipine (Cardene®) Verapamil (Calan®, Isoptin®, Verelan®)
Xanthine bronchodilators	Theophylline (Marax®, Quibron® etc.*)
Beta-adrenergic drugs (bronchodilators, anti-shock drugs)	Dopamine (from metabolism of Levodopa, but not from Sinemet®), Isoproterenol (Isuprel®), Ephedrine
Nitrates (oral, sublingual, or applied to the skin) for cardiac conditions	Deponit®, Dilatrate®, Imdur®, Ismo®, Isordil®, Monoket®, Nitro-Bid®, Nitrodisc®, Nitro-Dur®, Sorbitrate®, Transderm-Nitro®
Steroid anti-inflammatory drugs, hormones	Corticosteroids,* Anabolic steroids (Android® etc.), Progesterone

*For a list of common examples, see "Prescription Medicines That Often Cause Dyspepsia."

Sources and Resources

Lifestyle Management

Be Here Now, Ram Dass, Crown, New York, 1971.

Breaking Free of the Co-Dependency Trap, Barry K. Weinhold and Janae B. Weinhold, Stillpoint Publishing, Walpole, NH, 1989.

Co-Dependent No More, Melodie Beatty, Harper & Row, New York, 1987.

Dr. Dean Ornish's Program for Reversing Heart Disease, Chapters 5–9, "Opening Your Heart." Dean Ornish, Ballantine Books, New York, 1990.

Each Day a New Beginning; A Book of Daily Meditations for Women, Hazelden Meditation Series, Hazelden Educational Materials, Center City, MN, 1982.

Freedom though Higher Awareness, Wayne W. Dyer, Nightingale-Conant Corporation, 1996. 1-800-323-5552 (audiotape series).

Full Catastrophe Living: Using the Wisdom of Your Body and Mind to Face Stress, Pain, and Illness, Jon Kabat-Zinn, Delta, New York, 1991.

Habits Not Diets, 3rd ed., James M. Ferguson and Cassandra Ferguson, Bull Publishing Co., Palo Alto, CA 1997.

Healing Sounds: The Power of Harmonics, Jonathan Goldman, Element, Inc., Rockport, MA, 1992.

Integral Yoga has centers in most cities: 1-800-858-YOGA for information, or iyi@yogaville.org.

Kripalu Yoga has trained over 5,000 yoga teachers worldwide: 1-413-448-3202 or www.kripalu.org.

Living Arts yoga videos: Yoga Practice for Beginners with Patricia Walden; Yoga Practice for Flexibility with Patricia Walden; Yoga Practice for Relaxation with Patricia Walden and Rodney Yee. 1-800-254-8464 or www.livingarts.com.

Peace Is Every Step: The Path of Mindfulness in Everyday Life, Thich Nhat Hanh, Bantam Books, New York, 1991.

Recent Experience Scale, Thomas H. Holmes, MD, Department of Psychiatry and Behavioral Sciences, University of Washington School of Medicine, Seattle, WA 98195.

The Relaxation Response, Herbert Benson, Morrow, New York, 1975.

The Secrets to Manifesting Your Destiny, Wayne W. Dyer, Nightingale-Conant Corporation, 1994. 1-800-323-5552 (audiotape series).

Sounds of Healing, Mitchell L. Gaynor, M.D., Broadway Books, New York, 1999.

"Stress," Jerry Adler, *Newsweek*, June 8, 1999. Stress hormones increase in seconds to minutes after even tiny stresses.

Touchstones; A Book of Daily Meditations for Men, Hazelden Meditation Series, Hazelden Educational Materials, Center City, MN, 1986.

Wherever You Go, There You Are: Mindfulness Meditation in Everyday Life. Jon Kabat-Zinn, Hyperion, New York, 1994.

Yoga the Iyengar Way. Silva, Mira and Shyam Mehta, Alfred A. Knopf, New York, 1990.

The Yoga Site (www.yogasite.com) lists yoga teachers.

You'll See It When You Believe It, Wayne Dyer, HarperCollins, New York, 1990.

MEDICAL APPROACHES TO HEARTBURN, ULCER, GASTRITIS, AND ESOPHAGEAL REFLUX DISEASE

American College of Gastroenterology hotline, 800-HRT-BURN (478-2876) or fax to 703-931-4520. Offers a free fact sheet, a brochure, even a list of nearby gastroenterologists who belong to the college (this means they are board-certified in this subspecialty).

"Chronic Heartburn, an Ominous Warning," Jane E. Brody, *New York Times*, April 29, 1999. The risks of continuing heartburn include esophageal cancer.

"Dietary fatty acids are also drugs," Andrew J. Dannenberg and Marcus M. Reidenberg, Clinical Pharmacology and Therapeutics, Volume 55, pages 5–9, 1994. Reprint requests: Andrew Dannenberg, MD, Rm F-231, The New York Hospital-Cornell Medical Center, 1300 York Ave., New York, NY 10021.

"Efficacy of intensive dietary therapy alone or combined with lovastatin in outpatients with hypercholesterolemia," Donal B. Hunninghake, Evan A. Stein, et al., *New England Journal of Medicine*, Volume 328, 1993, pages 1213–1219. Reprint requests: Dr. Hunninghake, Heart Disease Prevention Clinic, 151 Variety Club Heart & Research Center, 401 E. River Rd., Minneapolis, MN 55455. Cutting dietary fat from 41% to 26% reduced cholesterol by only 5%.

"Fish consumption and the 30-year risk of fatal myocardial infarction," Martha L. Daviglus, Jeremiah Stamler, et al., *New England Journal of Medicine*, Volume 336, pages 1046–1052, 1997. More than 5 ounces twice a week gave maximum benefit. Reprint requests: Dr. Daviglus, Department of Preventive Medicine, Northwestern University Medical School, 680 North Lake Shore Dr., Suite 1102, Chicago IL 60611.

Gastroesophageal Reflux Disease (GERD), pamphlet, 1997, Krames Communications, San Bruno, CA. 1-800-333-3032 or ask your doctor for a copy.

Gastrointestinal Health, Steven Peikin, HarperCollins Publishers, New York, 1991.

Good Food for Bad Stomachs, Henry D. Janowitz, M.D., Oxford University Press, New York, 1997.

"Gut Reactions," Wendy Marston with Mary Hager, *Newsweek*, November 17, 1997. Too much aspirin, ibuprofen, alcohol, or antibiotics can cause leaks in the lining of the small intestine and cause asthma, arthritis, fatigue, food allergies, etc.

Harrison's Principles of Internal Medicine, 8th ed., George W. Thorn, Raymond D. Adams, Eugene Braunwald, Kurt J. Isselbacher, and Robert G. Petersdorf, Blakiston, New York, 1977. Gastroenterology just before the anti-acid drugs.

Herbal medicine, Prescriber's Letter Document #131033, 1996. 1-209-472-2240 for information or fax 1-209-472-2249.

Physician's Desk Reference, 53rd ed., Health Economics, Montvale, NJ, 1999.

The Ulcer Story: The Authoritative Guide to Ulcers, Dyspepsia, and Heartburn, W. Grant Thompson, M.D., Plenum Press, New York, 1996.

HERBAL AND OTHER NATURAL APPROACHES

Fats That Heal, Fats That Kill, Udo Erasmus, Alive Books, Burnaby BC, Canada, 1993.

Heartburn and What to Do about It: A Guide to Overcoming the Discomforts of Indigestion Using Drug-Free Remedies, James F. Balch and Morton Walker, Avery Publishing Group, Garden City Park, New York, 1998.

The Herbal Guide and Handbook, Henry Hunt, Desert Press, Arizona City, AZ 1994.

"Herb News," Varro E. Tyler, *Prevention*, July 1999.

Joy of Cooking, Irma S. Rombauer and Marion Rombauer Becker, Plume, New York, 1973. A great resource, but don't use it for proportions of fats!

Mediterranean Light; Delicious Recipes from the World's Healthiest Cuisine, Martha Rose Shulman, Bantam Books, New York, 1989. Hold the onions, garlic, and peppers!

Prescription for Dietary Wellness, Phyllis A. Balch and James F. Balch, PAB Books, Inc., Greenfield, IN, 1993.

Prescription for Nutritional Wellness, James F. Balch and Phyllis A. Balch, Avery Publishing Group, Garden City Park, NY, 1990.

"Soy Cooking," Ruth Adams, *Better Nutrition for Today's Living*, March 1995. This monthly magazine is available free at many health food stores. 404-618-0385.

Stomach Ailments and Digestive Disturbances, Michael T. Murray, Prima Publishing, Rocklin, CA, 1997.

Stomach Ulcers: Safe Alternatives without Drugs, Leonard Mervyn, Thorsons Natural Health, HarperCollins Publishers, London, 1997.

Sunset Low-Fat Cookbook, Sunset Publishing Corporation, Menlo Park, CA, 1992.

"Ten Best Healing Herb Teas," Laura Goldstein, *Prevention,* April 1999.

GASTROENTEROLOGY LITERATURE

Alpers, David H. Why Should Psychotherapy Be a Useful Approach to Management of Patients With Nonulcer Dyspepsia? *Gastroenterology 2000*;119:869–871.

Fisher, R.S., and H.P. Parkman. Current Concepts: Management of Nonulcer Dyspepsia. *New England Journal of Medicine;* 339, November 5, 1998, 1376–1381.

Graham, David Y. Therapy of Helicobacter pylori: Current Status and Issues. *Gastroenterology 2000*;118:S2–S8.

Hamilton, Jane, Elspeth Guthrie, Francis Creed, et al. A Randomized Controlled Trial of Psychotherapy in Patients with Chronic Functional Dyspepsia. *Gastroenterology 2000*;119:661–669.

Hawkey, Chrisopher J. Nonsteroidal Anti-inflammatory Drug Gastropathy. *Gastroenterology 2000*;119:521–535.

Klinkenberg-Knol, Elly C., Frits Nelis, John Dent, et al. Long-Term Omeprazole Treatment in Resistant Gastroesophageal Reflux Disease: Efficacy, Safety, and Influence on Gastric Mucosa. *Gastroenterology 2000*:118:661–669.

Miwa, Takeshi, Ed. Dyspepsia: What's New? *Clinical Therapeutics;* 20, Supp. D, 1998. Excerpta Medica, Inc., Belle Mead, NJ. Reprint requests: Vicki Donoso, 1-908-281-3694.

Pandolfino, John E., Colin W. Howden, and Peter J. Kahrilas. Motility-Modifying Agents and Management of Disorders of Gastrointestinal Motility. *Gastroenterology 2000*;118:S32–S47.

Pope, Charles E., II. Acid Reflux Disorders. *New England Journal of Medicine;* 331, 656–660, 1994. Reprint requests: Dr. Pope, Division of Gastroenterology RG-24, University of Washington, Seattle, WA 98195. Esophageal reflux can even cause acid laryngitis with hoarseness, dry cough, etc.

Wolfe, M. Michael, and George Sachs. Acid Suppression: Optimizing Therapy for Gastroduodenal Ulcer Healing, Gastroesophageal Reflux Disease, and Stress-Related Erosive Syndrome. *Gastroenterology 2000*;118:S9–S31.

$\mathcal{I}$NDEX

Progressive relaxation, 52-53
Prokinetic drugs to help stomach, 247
Protein factor, 79-82
 amino acids, essential, 79-80
 what is needed and what is not,
  80-82
 glycemic index, 80-82
Proton pump inhibitors, 246
Psychodynamic-interpersonal therapy
  (PI), 36, 47, 48-49
Psychotherapy and stress management,
  35
Punch, 124
Ptyalin, 65

R

Ranch salad dressing, 158
Raspberry vinaigrette salad dressing,
  159
Rebound hyperacidity, 7
Recent Experience Scale, 40-43
Red potatoes, boiled, 186
Reflux:
 esophagitis, 244
 fluids as cause of, 30
Reglan®, 247
Relaxation Response, 51, 59
Relaxation for stress management, 36,
  51-61
 alpha waves, 51
 books, 54
  *Dr. Dean Ornish's Program for
   Reversing Heart Disease,* 54
  Yoga the Iyengar Way, 54
 deep muscle relaxation, 52-53
 hatha yoga, 51, 53-56
 meditation, 56-59
  distraction, dealing with, 57-58
  fundamentals, 57
  readings, 59
  transcendental, 57-58
  trip meditation, 60-61
 Mindfulness Meditation, 51, 58-59
 prayer, 59-60
 progressive relaxation, 52-53
 Relaxation Response, 51, 59

yoga classes, 53-56
 asanas, 54, 55
 *pose of the dead (corpse pose,
  savasana),* 55
yoga videos, 54
Rice, 16, 191-206
 brown, 192
 chicken portobello Belle, 204-205
 Chinese menu of stir-fried meat and
  vegetable recipes, 198-206
 and hearty greens, 194-196
 mushroom risotto, easy, 192-193
 rice erroneous, 193-194
 shopping for and storage of, 109
 stuffing, Jim's, 205-206
 un-garian lecso, 196-197
 veggie stir-fry bake, 202-203
 white, 191
 wild, 192
Ron's chicken Vesuvio, 211-212
Rosemary, 25
Running not advised, 18
Russet potatoes, baked, 186-187
Rye bread, making in breadmaker, 166

S

Sage, 26
Salads for lunch, 144 (*see also* Lunch)
Salad dressings, 156-161
 Babe's blue cheese, 160
 bacon, 158
  hot, 158-159
 blueberry or raspberry vinaigrette,
  159
 celery seed, 157-158
 honey mustard yogurt, 157
 Italian, 160-161
 making your own, 156
 ranch, 158
Salade nicoise Pacific Northwest style,
  150-151
Saliva, 65-66
Salmon, 104
 broiled with herbs, 212-214
 dip, 188-189, 207-208
 spread, hot, with hash browns, 189

ABOUT THE AUTHOR

Rob Pyke, M.D., Ph.D., is a specialist in clinical pharmacology and internal medicine who has directed clinical research on stomach acidity, ulcers, gastritis, irritable bowel syndrome, colitis, cardiovascular disease, and stress-related disorders. In 1994, after suffering severe erosive gastritis and gastroesophogeal reflux disease, Dr. Pyke began self-treatment, testing alternative and holistic approaches on himself. His thoroughly researched methods, and his holistic approach, led to full recovery.